29.99

Challenges and Solutions: Narratives of Patient-Centered Care

This book is due for return on or before the last date shown below.

Challenges and Solutions: Narratives of Patient-Centered Care

Edited by

JUDITH BELLE BROWN, Ph.D.
Professor, Centre for Studies in Family Medicine
Department of Family Medicine
Schulich School of Medicine and Dentistry
The University of Western Ontario

TANYA THORNTON, M.D., CCFP, M.Cl.Sc.(FM)
Adjunct Professor of Family Medicine
Department of Family Medicine
Schulich School of Medicine and Dentistry
The University of Western Ontario

and

MOIRA STEWART, Ph.D.
Professor, Centre for Studies in Family Medicine
Department of Family Medicine
Schulich School of Medicine and Dentistry
The University of Western Ontario

Radcliffe Publishing
London • New York

Radcliffe Publishing Ltd
33–41 Dallington Street
London
EC1V 0BB
United Kingdom

www.radcliffepublishing.com

British Library Cataloguing in Publication Data

A catalogue record for this book is available from the British Library.

ISBN-13: 978 184619 496 2

The paper used for the text pages of this book is FSC
certified. FSC (The Forest Stewardship Council)
is an international network to promote responsible
management of the world's forests.

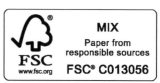

Typeset by KnowledgeWorks Global Ltd, Chennai, India
Printed and bound by TJI Digital, Padstow, Cornwall, UK

Contents

About the Editors

Judith Belle Brown, Ph.D., earned her degree in social work from Smith College, Northampton, MA, and is a professor in the Centre for Studies in Family Medicine, the Department of Family Medicine, Schulich School of Medicine and Dentistry at The University of Western Ontario (UWO), and in the School of Social Work at King's University College, London, Ontario, Canada. She is the Chair of the Masters in clinical science (M.Cl.Sc.) and Ph.D. programs in family medicine at UWO, both of which are offered via distance education. She has been conducting research on the patient-centered clinical method for over three decades. Dr. Brown has presented papers and conducted workshops both nationally (Canada and the United States) and internationally (UK, Holland, Spain, Hong Kong, Sweden, New Zealand, Australia, Denmark, Argentina, Brazil, Japan) on the patient-centered method. She is the co-author of *Patient-Centered Medicine: transforming the clinical method* and is a series editor along with Moira Stewart and Thomas R. Freeman of the following books: *Substance Abuse: a patient-centered approach; Chronic Fatigue Syndrome: a patient-centered approach; Chronic Myofascial Pain: a patient-centered approach; Eating Disorders: a patient-centered approach; Patient-Centred Prescribing: seeking concordance in practice; Palliative Care: a patient-centered approach; and Pregnancy and Childbirth: a woman-centered approach.*

She has also published papers dealing with patient-doctor communication in *Social Science & Medicine; Family Practice: an international journal; Patient Education and Counseling; Canadian Family Physician; and Journal of Family Practice.* Dr. Brown was a co-recipient of the American Academy on Physician and Patient Award for Outstanding Research in 1996. In the same year, Dr. Brown was made an Honorary Member of the College of Family Physicians of Canada. She was a co-recipient of the College of Family Physicians of Canada Best Original Research Article Award (2009) and the Dean's Award of Excellence – Team Award for the Centre for Studies in Family Medicine, the Schulich School of Medicine and Dentistry, The University of Western Ontario (2010).

Tanya Thornton, M.D., CCFP, M.Cl.Sc.(FM), graduated from medicine at the University of Toronto and completed postgraduate training, a fellowship in academic medicine and graduate studies at The University of Western Ontario (UWO). She is an adjunct professor of family medicine in the Schulich School of Medicine and Dentistry at The University of Western Ontario, London, Ontario, Canada, and practices comprehensive rural family medicine in St. Marys, Ontario. She was Clerkship Director, Department of Family Medicine, the Schulich School of Medicine and Dentistry, The University of Western Ontario from 2006 to 2008. Dr. Thornton has a special interest in both narrative writing and the patient-family physician relationship and has conducted research on how the electronic medical record affects the patient-family physician relationship (2006). Dr. Thornton teaches at UWO at the undergraduate, postgraduate and masters levels and was recipient of the 2011 Undergraduate Teacher of the Year for Family Medicine Award.

Moira Stewart, Ph.D., is a professor in the Centre for Studies in Family Medicine at The University of Western Ontario. She holds the Dr. Brian W. Gilbert Tier 1 Canada Research Chair in Primary Health Care Research. Dr. Stewart has published widely on the topic of patient-centered care and has edited with Judith Belle Brown and Thomas R. Freeman an international series of books applying the patient-centred clinical method. Dr. Stewart is a research methodologist, advocating for a wide variety of research methodologies in primary care. She was part of a team that sponsored five international symposia and edited five widely used books in a series called Foundations of Primary Care Research. She is the principal investigator on a strategic training grant on interdisciplinary primary health care research called TUTOR-PHC. This program has educated 91 researchers from more than eight disciplines across Canada. Dr. Stewart is also the principal investigator on the DELPHI (Deliver Primary Healthcare Information) project, creating a researchable database of the Electronic Medical Record data of 25 family physicians in Southwestern Ontario. In a new Applied Health Research Network Initiative (AHRNI), Dr. Stewart is the leader of the System Integration and Innovation Research Network (SIIReN) as well as the Primary Health Care System (PHCS). Dr. Stewart is an honorary member of the College of Family Physicians of Canada (1991). She received the James Mackenzie Medal of the Royal College of General Practitioners (2004), the College of Family Physicians of Canada Family Medicine Researcher of the Year Award (2007), and the Martin J. Bass Recognition Award, Department of Family Medicine, The University of Western Ontario (2008). She is also co-recipient of the Dean's Award of Excellence – Team Award for the Centre for Studies in Family Medicine at the Schulich School of Medicine & Dentistry, The University of Western Ontario, London, Ontario (2010), and she also holds a fellowship in the Canadian Academy of Health Sciences (2010).

List of Contributors

Dr. Ascia Hassan Abdi
Family Physician
Hargeisa, Somaliland

Dr. Sofian Al-Samak
Staff, Central Newfoundland Regional Health Centre
Grand Falls-Windsor, Newfoundland

Dr. Lemmese Al-Watban
Family Physician
Edmonton, Alberta

Dr. Rochelle Dworkin
Chief Obstetrics, Hanover and District Hospital
Family Physician, Hanover Medical Associates
Hanover, Ontario

Dr. Thomas R. Freeman
Family Physician and Chair
Department of Family Medicine
Schulich School of Medicine and Dentistry
The University of Western Ontario

Dr. Lisa Graves
Family Physician
Staff, Herzl Family Practice Centre, Sir Mortimer B. Davis Jewish General
Hospital
Assistant Professor, McGill University
Montreal, Quebec

Dr. Sharon Nur Hatcher
Family Physician
Associate Professor, Universite de Sherbrooke
Chicoutimi, Quebec

Dr. Hugh Hindle
Family Physician, Sylvan Family Health Centre
Sylvan Lake, Alberta

Dr. Nusrat Jamil
Family Physician, Broadview Medical Clinic
Broadview, Saskatchewan

Dr. Barbara Jones
Family Physician
Aitkenvale, Australia

Dr. Jill Konkin
Department of Family Medicine, University of Alberta
Edmonton, Alberta

Dr. Sudha Koppula
Family Physician, Royal Alexandra Hospital
Edmonton, Alberta

Dr. Barry Lavallee
Family Physician
Winnipeg, Manitoba

Dr. Joseph Lee
Family Physician, the Centre for Family Medicine
Kitchener, Ontario

Dr. Michael Lee-Poy
Assistant Clinical Professor, McMaster University
Adjunct Professor, The University of Western Ontario
Family Physician, Kitchener, Ontario

Dr. Michelle Levy
Family Physician, Grey Nuns Family Medicine Centre
Edmonton, Alberta

Dr. Sabrina Lim
Family Physician, Cambridge, Ontario

Dr. Peter MacKean
Family Physician
Summerside, PEI

Dr. Jana Malhotra
Family Physician, Nepean, Ontario

Dr. Carol L. McWilliam
Professor
School of Nursing
The University of Western Ontario

Dr. Bridget L. Ryan
Postdoctoral Fellow, Centre for Studies in Family Medicine, The University
of Western Ontario
London, Ontario

Dr. Larry Schmidt
Family Physician, St. Joseph's Family Medical and Dental Centre
Assistant Professor, Family Medicine, The University of Western Ontario
London, Ontario

Dr. Dori Seccareccia
Family Physician
Staff, Princess Margaret Hospital-University Health Network
Toronto, Ontario

Dr. Joshua Shadd
Assistant Professor, Family Medicine
Centre for Studies in Family Medicine, The University of Western Ontario
London, Ontario

Dr. Jeff Sisler
Director, Primary Care Oncology
Associate Professor, Family Medicine, University of Manitoba
CancerCare Manitoba
Winnipeg, Manitoba

Dr. Jane Uygur
Family Physician, Clairhurst Medical Centre
Toronto, Ontario

Dr. Adrienne Watson
Family Physician, Mayflower Medical Clinic
Halifax, Nova Scotia

Dr. W. Wayne Weston
Professor Emeritus, Family Medicine
The University of Western Ontario
London, Ontario

Dr. Eric Wong
Family Physician, St. Joseph's Family Medical and Dental Centre
London, Ontario

Dr. Susan Woolhouse
Family Physician, South Riverdale Community Health Centre
Toronto, Ontario

Acknowledgments

This book represents the accumulation of patient stories over a span of many years. Without question they are stories that challenge us and make us reflect on clinical practice. We are grateful to our colleagues, the authors of the narratives, who have been willing to share with us their experiences with patients, both positive and negative. We have also been inspired by the patients whose stories are reflected herein.

Sincere thanks is extended to Dr. Tom Freeman, Chair of the Department of Family Medicine, Schulich School of Medicine and Dentistry, The University of Western Ontario (from 1999–2011), for creating an environment that encouraged the time to teach, write and reflect.

We thank Andrea Burt for her outstanding coordination of this project. Her devotion and thoroughness has been exemplary. We also extend our thanks to Anne Fendrich, Sherry Benko and Magda Catani for their tolerance of our numerous edits and attention to detail.

Judith Belle Brown
Tanya Thornton
Moira Stewart
August 2011

Dedication

This book is dedicated to those health care providers who are committed to ensuring their patients receive optimal patient-centered care – care that preserves their patients' dignity and values both their health and illness experience. Every time a story is told, an emotion shared, a moment of vulnerability exposed, we are richer for it, and as such are enhanced in our ability to care and comfort those who are suffering.

Introduction

Stories capture us and take us on a journey. Sometimes they take us to a place that is familiar, resonates with our experience and hence reaffirms what we know and value. Other stories reveal experiences that are unknown to us and as such, may challenge our belief systems, beseeching us to wonder and reflect. Narratives about patients and their physicians continue to enrapture us, because at some time and point we will all be a patient. For physicians, narratives provide insight and illumination of what it truly means to be patient-centered. They also help clinicians to examine, in a reflective manner, what it means to be a healer.

Listening to stories, collecting stories, sharing stories and writing stories has been, in recent years, an important jewel in the practice and teaching of medicine. Authors from varied disciplines in medicine have passionately embraced the role of narratives, as they exquisitely detail the profound experiences of patients as well as the experiences of clinicians caring for those patients (Borkan *et al.* 1999; Brown *et al.* 2002; Cameron 2011; Charon 2004, 2006, 2007; Frank 1995, 2004; Greenhalgh and Hurwitz 1998; Groopman 2008; Nuland 2010; Ofri 2005).

For example, Rita Charon, an internationally renowned author on the power of narrative in medicine, explains: "More and more health care professionals and patients are recognizing the importance of stories they tell one another of illness." Charon contends that "only in the telling is the suffering made evident," and thus we must "accept our obligations to learn how to receive these stories" (NEJM 2004, p. 862).

Ian Cameron, a well-respected family physician and eloquent raconteur, asks: "Are narrative plot, words, the importance of listening, the importance of stories, and their values in the effective relationship between patients and doctors vital in the practice of medicine?" He then tells the following story: "I had a patient who, in his mid-50s, had a crisis of identity and purpose. I asked him to return in a week and tell me about his very first memories. He chronologically moved forward with his memories in 15-minute weekly sessions. By the sixth session, he had reconnected with his story and rediscovered himself" (CFP 2011, p. 67).

Jerome E. Groopman, in his forward to the book *Soul of a Doctor*, writes, "It has been said that all of literature can be divided into two themes: the first, a person goes on a journey; the second, a stranger comes to town. This is, of course, terribly simplistic, but there is a core of truth in it. And it is also true that narratives of medicine meld both these themes. A person goes on a journey: that person is the patient, but accompanying him on the voyage is the doctor. A stranger comes to town: that stranger is illness, the uninvited guest who disrupts the equilibrium of quotidian life. Where the journey leads, how the two voyagers change, and whether the stranger is ultimately expelled or in some way subdued give each narrative its unique drama" (Pories, Jain and Harper 2006, p. xi–xii).

Collectively, these authors value the place of narratives in medicine. Indeed, they would argue that narratives, or the patients' stories, are central to patient care. These stories are the essence of what we receive. We are privileged to bear witness to these stories and to sometimes be a part of them – from the beginning to the end.

This book presents examples of the many challenges encountered in patient-doctor interactions and provides some ideas for dealing with these problems more effectively. It does not address every concern, but it does highlight those common in day-to-day practice. What makes these narratives important and useful is that they are based on real situations – ones that we have all encountered and wondered how to handle. We hope to challenge you, to stimulate you to think, and most of all, to listen in a new and fruitful manner.

Overview of the Patient-Centered Clinical Method
For 30 years, the Centre for Studies in Family Medicine, Department of Family Medicine, Schulich School of Medicine and Dentistry, The University of Western Ontario has been developing and testing a method of practice that integrates the traditional medical model with a patient-centered approach endeavoring to understand the patient's unique experience of illness. A program of education, research and conceptual development led to a body of work represented in *Patient-Centered Medicine: transforming the clinical method* (2nd ed.), which described the six components (Stewart *et al.* 2003). The new and revised patient-centered clinical method is outlined below and consists of four interactive components to be considered in every patient-physician interaction.

Component I: Exploring Health, Disease and the Illness Experience
The first component involves exploring the patient's perceptions of health, disease and the illness experience. Primarily, health perceptions are the

person's sense of his or her own health and the benefits and barriers to that health. In addition to assessing the disease process by history and physical examination, the doctor explores the patient's illness experience. Specifically, the doctor considers how the patient feels about being ill, what the patient's ideas are about the illness, what impact the illness is having on the patient's functioning, and what he or she expects from the physician.

Component II: Understanding the Whole Person

The second component integrates the concepts of health, disease and illness with an understanding of the whole person. This includes an awareness of the patient's position in the life cycle and their proximal and distal contexts.

Component III: Finding Common Ground

The third component of the method is the process of finding common ground between the patient and the doctor. This consists of reaching a mutual understanding and a mutual agreement with regard to: defining the problem(s), examining the goals and priorities of treatment, and identifying the roles to be assumed by both the patient and the doctor.

Component IV: Enhancing the Patient-Doctor Relationship

The fourth component takes into consideration that each encounter with the patient should be used to develop the patient-doctor relationship. The trust and respect that evolves in the relationship will have an impact on other components of the method.

The Value of the Patient-Centered Clinical Method

There is strong evidence supporting the efficacy of patient-centered care, which has been associated with: higher patient satisfaction (Fossum and Arborelius 2004; Krupat *et al.* 2000; Stewart *et al.* 1999), better patient adherence (Golin *et al.* 1996; Stewart *et al.* 1999), better patient health outcomes such as reduction of concern and discomfort (Stewart *et al.* 2000), better self-reported health (Stewart *et al.* 2000; Stewart *et al.* 2007), improved physiological status, e.g. blood pressure, metabolic control for patients with diabetes, (Golin *et al.* 1996; Greenfield *et al.* 1988; Griffin *et al.* 2004; Kaplan *et al.* 1989; Krupat *et al.* 2000; Rao *et al.* 2007; Stewart *et al.* 1999); and lower costs of care (Epstein *et al.* 2005; Stewart *et al.* 2011). Furthermore, the patient-centered component of finding common ground has been associated with lower utilization of medical services (Stewart *et al.* 2000).

The patient-centered method is valuable to physicians for several reasons. First, the clinical method is a reasonable representation of the realities of medical practice. By providing a useful framework, the patient-centered clinical method guides physicians in their complex work of caring for patients. Because the method grew out of medical practice, it has immediate applicability by both novice as well as experienced physicians.

Second, the patient-centered method applies to the majority of interactions between patients and doctors. It is not geared only towards counseling or interviewing, but can be employed with patients of all ages with a variety of health issues and concerns.

Third, it describes what doctors do when they are functioning well with their patients; thus it supplies a conceptual framework for physicians in their daily practice. The patient-centered clinical method is more than an exhortation to be more caring; it describes specific behaviors that need to be learned, and it explains when and how to use them with patients. Because this clinical method is explicit about the behavior of an effective clinician, it also provides a vocabulary and a focus for teaching and learning.

About the Stories

The narratives presented in the first four sections of this book highlight each of the four components of the patient-centered clinical method. The stories in the fifth and final section illustrate how the enactment of patient-centered care requires attending to many, if not all, of the components that comprise the patient-centered clinical method. This reflects the interactive and dynamic nature of the patient-centered clinical method and emphasizes how clinicians must shift from one component of the method to another as they follow patients' cues. The analogy is to a dance: as one partner responds to the tempo and nuance of the music, the other follows, and then vice versa. The mutual rhythm that is created is influenced by the environment or context in which the "dance" or interaction transpires.

Several of the stories illustrated in this book reflect our aging population. This is not unexpected, as the care of this group of individuals may be our greatest clinical challenge in the future. Hopefully, these stories provide some guidance as to how we can best address the ever-growing demands for patient-centered care of this most valued cohort of patients. Another group of patients to which we extend a special focus are those who are disadvantaged and vulnerable. They are now desperately in need of our care.

While most of these narratives have been written from the perspective of family physicians, the basic tenets of patient-centered care are transferrable to all health care professionals who are committed to providing exemplary health care.

The names and many identifying characteristics of the individuals portrayed in the narratives have been changed to protect confidentiality. All of these stories are based on real experiences, most often described by physicians. In some instances, the stories have originated from patients', or family members', own personal experiences. From our perspective, these stories have tremendous validity and value; they exemplify the human qualities of suffering, conflict and perseverance. On many occasions, we are privileged to witness the patient's triumph over tragic and troubled circumstances. Time and time again, we see the critical role of communication in these triumphs. When we take time to listen – to give value to people's stories, their fears, their angst and their sorrow – we gain a deeper and more thorough appreciation of their suffering, and the listening ultimately provides direction in the process of healing.

COMPONENT I

Exploring Health, Disease and the Illness Experience

Moira Stewart, Judith Belle Brown,
W. Wayne Weston, Carol L. McWilliam and
Thomas R. Freeman

To practice patient-centered medicine, clinicians must explore three inter-related concepts: health, disease and illness. Effective patient care requires attending as much to patients' perceptions of health and personal experiences of illness as to their disease. Disease is diagnosed by using the conventional medical model, but understanding health and illness requires a different approach. Disease is diagnosed by objective observation; it is a category; the "thing" that is wrong with the body-as-machine or the mind-as-computer. Disease is a theoretical construct or abstraction by which physicians attempt to explain patients' problems in terms of abnormalities of structure and/or function of body organs and systems; it includes both physical and mental disorders. Illness, for its part, is the patient's personal and subjective experience of sickness; the feelings, thoughts and altered behavior of someone who feels sick. Health perceptions, for their part, are the person's sense of his or her own health and the benefits and barriers to it.

In the biomedical model, sickness is explained in terms of pathophysiology: abnormal structure and function of tissues and organs. This model is a conceptual framework for understanding the biological dimensions of sickness by reducing sickness to disease. The focus is on the body, not the person. A particular disease is what everyone with that disease has in common, but the health perceptions and illness experiences of each person are unique. Disease and illness do not always coexist; health and disease are not always mutually exclusive. Patients with undiagnosed, asymptomatic disease

perceive themselves to be healthy and do not feel ill; people who are grieving or worried may feel ill but have no disease. Patients and doctors who
recognize these distinctions and who realize how common it is to perceive
a loss of health or feel ill and yet have no disease are less likely to search
needlessly for pathology. However, even when disease is present, it may
not adequately explain the patient's suffering, since the amount of distress
a patient experiences refers not only to the amount of tissue damage but to
the personal meaning of health and illness.

Several authors have described these same interrelated concepts of
health, disease and illness from different perspectives. In analyzing medical
interviews, Mishler (1984) identifies contrasting voices: the voice of medicine and the voice of the lifeworld. The voice of medicine promotes a scientific, detached attitude and uses questions such as: "Where does it hurt?
When did it start? How long does it last? What makes it better or worse?"
The voice of the lifeworld, on the other hand, reflects a "common-sense"
view of the world. It centers on the individual's particular social context,
the meaning of health and illness, and how they may affect the achievement of personal health goals. Typical questions to explore the lifeworld
include: "How would you describe your health? What are you most concerned about? How does your loss of health disrupt your life? What do you
think it is? How do you make sense of what has happened to you? How do
you think I can help you?"

FOUR DIMENSIONS OF THE ILLNESS EXPERIENCE

We propose four dimensions of the illness experience that physicians should
explore: patients' feelings, especially their fears, about their problems; their
ideas about what is wrong; the effect of the illness on their functioning; and
their expectations of the clinician.

*What are the patients' **feelings**?* Do they fear that the symptoms they present may be the precursor of a more serious problem such as cancer? Some
patients may feel a sense of relief and view the illness as an opportunity for
relief from demands or responsibilities. Patients often feel irritated or cul-
pable about being ill.

*What are the patients' **ideas** about their illness?* On one level the patients'
ideas may be straightforward, e.g. "I wonder if these headaches could be
migraine headaches." But at a deeper level patients may struggle to find the
meaning of their illness experience. Many persons face illness as an irrepa-
rable loss; others may view it as an opportunity to gain valuable insight
into their life experience. Is the illness seen as a form of punishment, or

perhaps as an opportunity for dependency? Whatever the illness, knowing its meaning is significant for understanding the patient.

*What are the **effects of the illness on function**?* Does it limit patients' daily activities? Does it impair their family relationships? Does it require a change in lifestyle? Does it compromise their quality of life? Does the patient see any connection between his headaches and the guilty feelings he has been struggling with?

*What are their **expectations** of the doctor?* Does the presentation of a sore throat carry with it an expectation of an antibiotic? Do they want the doctor to take action or just listen? In a review and synthesis of the literature on patient expectations of the consultation, Thorsen *et al.* (2001) provide a further conceptualization of patients' expectations of the visit. They suggest that patients may come to a doctor visit with "a priori wishes and hopes for specific process and outcome" (p. 638). At times these expectations may not be explicit and, in fact, patients may modify or change their expectations during the course of the consultation.

The following examples of patient-clinician dialogue contain specific questions that physicians might ask to elicit this information.

To the doctor's question, "What brings you today?" a patient responds, "I've had these nagging headaches for the last few weeks. I'm wondering if there is something that I can do about them." The patient's feelings about the headaches can be elicited by questions such as: "What are your concerns about the headaches? Do you think that something specific is causing the pain? Is there something particularly worrisome for you about these headaches?"

To examine the patient's ideas about the headaches, the physician might ask (waiting after each question for the patient's reply): "What do you think is causing the pain? Have you any ideas or theories about why you might be having them? Do you think there is any relationship between your headaches and your current life situation? Most patients try to understand their problems on their own before coming to see me – by talking with family members or searching the Internet. Have you found out anything that you are wondering about?"

To determine how the headaches may be impeding the patient's function, the doctor might ask: "How are your headaches affecting your day-to-day living? Are they stopping you from participating in any activities? Is there any connection between your headaches and the way your life is going?"

Finally, to identify this particular patient's expectations of the physician at this visit, the doctor might inquire, "What do you think would help you to deal with these headaches? Is there some specific treatment that you want for your pain? In what way may I help you? Have you a particular test in mind? What do you think would reassure you about these headaches? Are you interested in medication for your headaches or do you primarily want to make sure they are not caused by something serious?"

Certain illnesses or events in the lives of individuals may cause them embarrassment or emotional discomfort. As a result, patients may not always feel at ease with themselves or their physician and may cloak their primary concerns in a myriad of symptoms. The doctor must, on occasion, respond to each of these symptoms to create an environment in which patients may feel more trusting and comfortable about exposing their concerns. Often, the doctor will provide them with an avenue to express their feelings by commenting: "I sense that there is something troubling you or something more is going on. How can I help you with that?" Finally, identifying the key questions to be asked should not be taken lightly. Malterud (1994), in describing a method for clinicians to formulate and evaluate the wording of key questions, emphasizes that the wording of questions should be comfortable for the doctor and suited to the patient's context.

DIMENSIONS OF HEALTH

In general, patients' definitions of health undoubtedly influence their life and their care. Also, the providers' definition of health, and their role in promoting health, inevitably permeates the care offered. Just as understanding the illness experience requires inquiry into feelings, ideas, effect on function and expectations, so too do health promotion and disease prevention strategies that are patient-centered. This includes an exploration of the individual's self-perceived health, perceptions of his or her susceptibility and seriousness of the disease, ideas about health promotion, and finally the perceived benefits and barriers to health promotion and prevention.

To practice patient-centered care, clinicians must think about the different conceptualizations of health as well as understand the patient's understanding (way of defining) health for him- or herself. Historically there have been three conceptualizations of health: 1) health has been understood to mean the absence of disease, and this meaning holds true within the biomedical model of clinical practice today; 2) in 1940, the World Health Organization (WHO 1986) defined health as "a state of complete mental, social and physical well-being, not merely the absence of disease and infirmity"; and 3) in 1986, the World Health Organization (WHO 1986) redefined health as "a resource for everyday life, not the objective of living," a concept of health that emphasizes social and personal resources as well as physical capacities.

Thus, the notion of health has shifted from its former abstract focus on physical, and then physical, mental and social status, toward "an ecological understanding of the interaction between individuals and their social and physical environment" (de Leeuw 1989; Hurowitz 1993; Stachtchenko and Jenicek 1990). While the earlier definitions direct attention to objective factual data, the most recent definition directs attention to the subjective and intersubjective experience and enactment of health. How patients and practitioners think about and, therefore, experience health continues to evolve. In fact, all partners in health care have unique and often differing understandings of health, and in turn, different understandings of health promotion and disease prevention to contribute to these aspects of health care.

In summary, the more favorable the patient's potential for health, particularly as it relates to self-efficacy and health status, the more appropriate the practitioner's role as facilitator of health enhancement and educator regarding risk avoidance. The less favorable the patient's potential for health, the more appropriate professional intervention will be with risk reduction and early identification strategies. Therefore, in disease prevention, as with health promotion, the practitioner's explicit recommendation is key. After that, understanding the patients' definition of health, their beliefs and attitudes and their past experiences will help the practitioner enhance health-promoting and disease-preventing behaviors (Pullen *et al.* 2001).

CONCLUSION

The first component of the patient-centered clinical method is the exploration of the patient's health, disease and unique illness experience. These three concepts can be considered individually or in various combinations, as they overlap with one another. In particular, it is important to elicit the four dimensions of the patient's illness experiences: their feelings, ideas, impact on function and expectations.

Preview of the Narratives

The following narratives illustrate how doctors explore the health, disease and unique illness experience of their patients.

We begin with a story depicting an individual suffering from symptoms that defy diagnosis. Failure to provide a label or diagnosis can be emotionally wearing for patients and cause undue suffering. Recognition of their illness experience and validation that their symptoms are real can be therapeutic and foster healthy coping.

In the second story, **Chapter 2**, we encounter a young woman transition-
ing from adolescence to adulthood. While she has escaped the terror of
her war-torn country, she cannot evade the all-encompassing sorrow of her
illness experience and the disease that will take her life away.

Chapter 3 serves as an example of how we often struggle to make sense
of the patient's illness experience – it is often hidden under an emotional
ice pack with layers depicting a complicated history and its subtle nuances.
Perhaps we cannot penetrate this solid stance or enter this frozen zone but
only respect and accept the patient's choices.

The fourth story, **Chapter 4**, recounts the narrative of a young man who
perceives himself as both healthy and a "rising star" in his work life. Yet, he
is plagued by a family legacy of depression, which shatters his self-esteem
and his perception of his health. While the onset of depression threatens his
equilibrium, the clinician assists him in not only accepting the diagnosis but
in making sense of his illness experience and ultimately regaining a sense of
health.

Living with a chronic illness can be emotionally wearing, as the
Chapter 5 narrative reveals. First, one must come to terms with the diagnosis and adjust life accordingly. But new opportunities and hopes for
the future can be threatened by an exacerbation of the disease process. A
patient-centered approach attends to the shifts and changes that are experienced by patients living with a chronic disease.

Sometimes an accidental event can uncover an incidental finding, as
Chapter 6 portrays. This narrative also underscores how one simple, and seemingly benign, life event can become an icon in the patient's illness experience.

The seventh and eighth narratives (**Chapter 7** and **Chapter 8**) are similar
in that both patients are confronted by a terminal disease. But for each individual, their illness experience is unique: one is a young mother, whose cancer will deprive her of the opportunity to witness the growth of her young
children; for the other woman, her rare disease shatters the relative "common" and gentle world in which she has existed.

The final two narratives, **Chapter 9** and **Chapter 10**, demonstrate how
two women suffer the same acute injury, a Colles' fracture of their left arm.
One woman is 19 years of age, the other is 70. While their diagnosis and
subsequent treatment are identical, their illness experiences are radically different. Their individual stories reveal how they exist in different worlds, and
decades far apart, despite the shared diagnosis. These narratives serve as a
transition to the next component of the patient-centered clinical method –
understanding the whole person.

*Narratives Illustrating Component I:
Exploring Health, Disease
and the Illness Experience*

1 Loss of Voice – Loss of Self

Michelle Levy, Judith Belle Brown and Tanya Thornton

It was my first day back after being on maternity leave. My inaugural patient was Silvia, a 51-year-old woman I had known for five years.

When I last saw Silvia a year ago, she had been experiencing a sore throat, hoarse voice and persistent cough for six weeks. We had tried standard treatments for a viral illness, allergies and allergic rhinitis with little success. At our last visit, Silvia expressed how she was finding it difficult to fulfill her role as a teacher. By the end of the workday, her voice had all but disappeared. "I am just so hoarse. I lose my voice. It's awful!" Silvia stated with exasperation. As I went off on my leave, I arranged for her to have a laryngoscopy with subsequent follow-up by the locum covering my practice.

Now one year later, in reviewing her chart, I read in detail everything that transpired during my absence. Silvia had attended the clinic for multiple visits. What I had viewed at the time as a self-limited or easily treatable problem had continued to intensify and was still without a clear diagnosis. Silvia's symptoms escalated. On a good day she could speak in a whisper. Her coughing episodes became more debilitating. "It is always worse in the morning," she explained wearily. "Sometimes it can take me one to two hours just to get up, shower and dress. Ventolin helps a little with my shortness of breath, but nothing helps with the cough."

In the past year, Silvia had been seen by multiple specialists, including a general internist, a respirologist, a neurologist, an otolaryngologist, a speech therapist and a psychotherapist. After extensive blood work, a laryngoscopy, a bronchoscopy, CT scans, pulmonary function tests and an MRI, there was still no real explanation for her ongoing symptoms, and no relief. While there were subtle findings on some tests, nothing was diagnostic. She was given a provisional diagnosis of functional aphonia and questionable asthma.

Silvia's entire life had changed. Previously employed as a teacher, she was now unable to work. On most days she could speak no louder than a whisper. Although Silvia had continued with speech therapy, which at times alleviated her symptoms, she would inevitably plateau or relapse. A one-time avid athlete, she now exercised only as tolerated. And of course, she went to medical appointments. With no clear diagnosis, but some "soft signs" on various tests, she continued the round of follow-up visits with the specialists and repeated testing every 3–6 months.

My attention returned to Silvia, sitting before me. In exasperation, she recounted her last visit with the general internist, who had raised the possibility of depression contributing to her symptoms. "I feel like they are all giving up on me, that it's all just in my mind," she said despondently. Silvia explained that during her visit with the internist, she became frustrated and tearful by her entire situation.

"Do you think you are depressed, Silvia?" I asked.

Her head jerked upward and our eyes locked. With a piercing glare she asserted, "Oh, I am very frustrated by these unexplainable symptoms! My life is extremely limited now and I find that very upsetting. But I am not depressed. If anything, I'm more worried that we don't get any answers!" There was no question in her mind that how she was feeling was the result of what was going on, not the cause.

"What worries you the most?" I asked gently.

"It's just the not knowing," Silvia replied, her eyes filling with tears.

As we discussed her situation further, Silvia described how she would almost prefer to learn that she had some terrible disease, just so there might be a treatment, or at least an understanding of what would transpire in the future. Without a diagnosis, no one really understood what she was experiencing – not her friends, not her family, not her previous employer, nor the disability company. And now she felt, maybe not even her health care providers. Silvia felt disconnected from those around her who had no comprehension of her suffering. It was a lonely existence.

Prompted by her psychotherapy sessions, Silvia began reflecting. She pondered how her future months and years would unfold. Silvia had come to realize that she was probably never going to be able to teach again. Nor would she be able to exercise as she had done in the past. There would be no more hiking trips with her 20-year-old son, no long walks in the evening with her husband. She wasn't really sure who she was anymore. "I've not only lost my voice, but I fear I am losing myself," whispered Silvia, her voice faint and weary. As I sat there listening, it occurred to me that Silvia was almost describing word for word the illness experience of a patient without a definable disease: the frustration of not knowing, the isolation from previous supports, the sense of disconnection, the loss of self.

On further discussion, what Silvia really wanted was a "game plan." Silvia had come to the realization that whatever was going on was not about to resolve quickly. "So I just need to learn to live with it," she said with conviction. Silvia demonstrated remarkable insight into her situation and viewed the psychotherapy sessions as key to her coping. She was coming to terms with the knowledge that she would never teach again and was actively exploring other employment options that wouldn't rely on her voice. Silvia explained how she was trained and certified in general accounting. Although she hadn't practiced for years, and would need to retake some exams, it was a career she both excelled at and enjoyed.

Finally, we discussed Silvia's expectations and the next steps regarding her medical visits. She would be following up in three months with her internist, who would repeat the CT chest and pulmonary function tests. At that point, she would also have an appointment with the respirologist for a CT scan; if the still showed some inflammation, the respirologist would consider a lung biopsy. In the meantime, Silvia was keen to continue meeting with her psychotherapist and to see me monthly to help coordinate her care. In the end, Silvia admitted she felt "better able to cope" and "more in control." Although still frustrated and unsure how to deal with those who doubted her symptoms were real, Silvia was optimistic that she would be able to find new employment and activities to replace those she sacrificed.

This case highlights how patients struggle to cope when suffering an illness without a definitive disease. When a diagnosis is not readily forthcoming, patients may become increasingly frustrated and start to question themselves as to whether it is "all in my head." This can be exacerbated by others who voice similar doubts – family, friends, employers and health care providers. Patients may believe that an actual diagnosis would be a tremendous relief, even if frightening, just to know what the "disease" is and to affirm that they are "not going crazy." The sense of disconnectedness and loss of self can be profound and prompt existential inquiry, such as: "Who am I now that I am sick?" This case also illustrates that exploring the patient's illness experience, while not solving the physical symptoms, can be beneficial in terms of alleviating fears, helping the patient to cope with the experience of illness and by imparting more control over her journey of suffering.

2 The Lonely Journey with Lupus

Ascia Hassan Abdi and Judith Belle Brown

"I can't believe that I'm in a hospital and dying. I have been diagnosed with systematic lupus erythematosus. I never thought this would happen to me, I never included it in my plans." Noria paused briefly to stop the tears that were running down her cheeks. "The internist talked to me openly," she continued. "He told me, 'The disease is pursuing a virulent course, leading to serious impairment of the kidneys.' I can't bear to think of myself on a dialysis machine for the rest of my life." Noria sobbed uncontrollably. Her eyes filled up with grief and horror. I reached out and touched her hand. In my mind I was thinking that this moment was one of those times when even the most empathetic words would have little effect on a patient. Maybe just listening could somehow ease her suffering.

Noria had just turned 18 years old. Along with her mother and sister, she moved to Canada four years ago because of the civil war in her native country. Noria recalled the brutality of the war, the loss of so many relatives and friends. She did not know her father's whereabouts. The last time she saw him was a morning in May, when he dropped her off at school. Noria waved goodbye as usual, thinking that she was going to see him at suppertime. That was their last contact before she left her country. After much hardship, Noria reached Canada, where she adapted quite well to her new environment. She learned the English language easily and made many friends. Sometimes I saw Noria in the mall near my office, chatting and "hanging out" with her friends, laughing at everything like so many teens of her age.

When I went to visit her the following day at the hospital, she looked thin and worn. Noria gazed at me with empty eyes. When I asked her how she was feeling, Noria answered me in a soft voice, "Not well, but I am glad to see you. You are my doctor; maybe you can explain to me some of the words that the internist told me about my disease."

Her doctor had explained to Noria that she had systematic lupus erythematosus (SLE). For her this was just a long name, with an even longer list of complications. I explained to her that this was an idiopathic autoimmune disease affecting multiple organs. The only thing Noria could really comprehend was that this disease was killing her. The tears streamed down her cheeks. She was anxious and there was desperation in her voice. Noria was confused and unable to manage the details. She had never heard of anyone in her family who had this disease before. "I am trying to understand why it chose me? Why it waited for my eighteenth birthday? Why couldn't it have happened maybe a little later in my life?" She paused to rest a few minutes, and then her anger and frustration was revealed. "This disease has cancelled all of my aspirations, dreams, hopes and happiness. I am in a new world, the world of the sick, the world of illness, the world of pain and suffering."

Noria's anger and desperation was palpable. I let her talk and talk without interruption, just nodding. I was feeling a bit helpless myself and felt at a loss to provide any meaningful advice or words of comfort to soothe her pain, which was apparent at multiple levels.

In the next days, when I visited her at the hospital, she was becoming more depressed and withdrawn, with little interest in life. In addition, Noria had developed debilitating joint pain in her hands that was resistant to analgesia. In the ensuing days, the pain intensified. I suggested that she talk to her joints, as they were listening. At first, Noria dismissed this, saying that it was "a crazy idea." She doubted such activity could have much effect. On second thought, since no other treatment was helping, Noria agreed to try it. She began daily conversations with her joints. Noria started talking about all the good times they had experienced together as a whole body, without problems, living in harmony. She recalled how she used to listen to music, dance, go for walks with her friends or spend long hours on Facebook hanging out with friends. Now she was too weak to talk, to walk. To move even a "finger" was an excruciatingly painful process.

Noria explained that sometimes even *thinking* was an exhausting process. On alternate days, she received dialysis for at least seven hours. On the Dialysis Unit she made some new friends, those with end-stage kidney disease, like herself. Noria doubted that her old friends would ever understand why she embraced these new friends, nor would they ever understand how much she shared with them and the deep comfort they provided during this difficult time. These new friends were in the same situation, the same world of despair and solitude. They shared the same hope of waiting and wishing that their disease would vanish the next day, a day that would never come.

The following week when I visited Noria, she talked about how she did not like to answer the telephone, or to see anyone. Painfully, Noria described how she did not feel that she had any connection with her previous friends or past life. She did not want pity. Instead, she wanted everyone to remember her the way she was before: healthy, happy and with a smile for everyone. She told me, "I am comforted in my bed. It gives me a hug of welcome back. I am able to ease my pain a little bit by lying down. I feel I am 90 years old, with arthritis in all my joints and uncontrollable blood pressure. My kidneys are on dialysis and I am all puffy with edema." Noria sighed deeply and continued, "The scary part of the disease is to feel so alone in the dreadful and helpless journey of this illness. It is a journey that you do not wish any companion ... I do not want anyone to suffer as I am. I want to say more, about the pain of mine but ... tomorrow is another fight between lupus and me. I have to spare some energy for the next battle. The war is not over yet. But I am glad you are here with me." In this precious moment we both smiled, and I experienced a surge of compassion for Noria, along with a ray of hope.

I have always believed that a patient's role is to tell the physician what hurts, and the physician's role is to fix it. But during this journey with Noria and her illness, she gave me much more than I had given her. She gave me her grateful heart, a chance to enhance my self-awareness and at the same time have a broader understanding of the task of medicine. I no longer feel uncomfortable in expressing compassion and understanding toward the suffering of a fellow human being nor of being patient-centered in the truest sense of the definition.

3 Frozen

Joshua Shadd

Dr. Parvinder caught himself sighing as he walked slowly down to the clinic. He remembered hearing someplace about "heartsink" patients – the patients whose names made your heart sink as soon as you saw them on your appointment list. Although he had met her only once, this described his reaction to Mrs. Gregor perfectly.

Dr. Parvinder's only previous meeting with Mrs. Gregor was six months earlier – when, like now, he was covering for her usual physician. It was an appointment he remembered clearly. Hers was a memorable story. Five years earlier, at the age of 69, she had been diagnosed with breast cancer. Following a lumpectomy, it was recommended that she undergo adjuvant radiation or chemotherapy. The idea of these cancer therapies terrified her, and she decided against them, holding onto the thin hope that surgery alone had been curative. Eighteen months later, she developed back pain. Eighteen more months passed before she mentioned this to her physician. The X-rays seemed like a formality. The foreshadowing was too strong: metastatic breast cancer. There would, of course, be no chemotherapy.

Since then, she has been haunted by a never-ending combination of symptoms that, for her, were deeply intertwined. Pain. Nausea. Difficulty swallowing. Fatigue. All of these symptoms fluctuating constantly and unpredictably. None responding more than marginally to anything her doctors offered. And all wrapped up in several layers of the anxiety and depression that had plagued her since the birth of her second daughter nearly five decades ago.

All of this ran through Dr. Parvinder's mind as he flipped through her chart before entering the room. Perusing his colleague's recent notes, it was apparent that little had changed since their first encounter. A recent CT scan showed stable disease. Medications for pain and nausea had been adjusted up, then down, then up again. He was disappointed, though not surprised, to read that she had not followed through with the psychiatry referral that he had made for her six months ago. He knew that today's appointment would not be short, and it would not change anything.

He put on a gentle smile and entered the room. Mrs. Gregor mumbled hello, but did not meet his gaze. She behaved as though she were trying to avoid disturbing the air. Dr. Parvinder was relieved that she did not look acutely ill. In fact, she looked no different than she had half a year ago. Mr. Gregor, a retired military officer, rose and shook Dr. Parvinder's hand firmly. He was a faithful companion at each of her appointments.

The three settled into familiar roles, with Dr. Parvinder listening attentively as Mrs. Gregor described her symptoms and Mr. Gregor occasionally interjecting with his observations. When Mrs. Gregor commented on how difficult she was finding it to cope with everything, Dr. Parvinder took the opportunity to ask about the psychiatry referral. For the first time that afternoon, Mrs. Gregor did not reply. After a pause, her husband responded on her behalf, and said in a surprisingly frosty tone, "Let's just assume everything from the neck up is taken care of, okay?" Dr. Parvinder, understanding that there would be no common ground on that issue today, moved on to another topic. He feared that he was implicitly endorsing a destructively false mind/body dichotomy by asking about her pain without discussing her suffering, but what could he do? His colleague's notes made it plain that she shared the same frustration: everything from the neck up was clearly *not* taken care of, and hadn't been for a long time.

During his initial visit with Mrs. Gregor, she told him about when she last felt well. It had been 10 years ago, when she was given a combination of antidepressant medications by a "psychiatrist who made me laugh." Then they moved. First to a new city for her husband's work, then across the country to where her younger daughter lives, and then to yet another city where her eldest daughter lives. The same medications prescribed by other doctors never seemed to do the trick.

Her support system was quite thin. As a military family, they had always moved often, and that pattern evidently continued into retirement. She had acquaintances all over the country, but no close friends. Her daughters were supportive but had families of their own. Her husband was her stalwart, but he openly acknowledged his frustration at the intractable nature of her suffering and the toll that this was taking on him. In fact, Dr. Parvinder was somewhat taken aback by Mr. Gregor's frank tone. "Dr. Parvinder, I can't tell you what a strain all of this has been on me. I'm sick of it all. I love my wife dearly, but there are days when I really feel at the end of my rope!"

Almost an hour later, Dr. Parvinder walked out of the examining room. He had assessed each of her symptoms in detail, asking her questions she had answered literally a thousand times before. They had reviewed options – more tests, new medications, more of the old medications. Mrs. Gregor didn't hold much optimism for any of these, and frankly neither did Dr. Parvinder. In the end, Mrs. Gregor said she preferred to leave everything unchanged.

She's stuck, thought Dr. Parvinder as he scribbled a note in the chart. She has moved many times, but she's been stuck for 50 years.

Then he changed his mind. No, not stuck. Stuck implies an attempt to move that is externally constrained. Mrs. Gregor isn't attempting to move or change. If anything, she seemed to be trying not to. "*She isn't stuck,*" thought Dr. Parvinder, "*she's frozen. I wish I could have helped her to begin to unfreeze.*"

Mrs. Gregor was still on his mind as Dr. Parvinder climbed into bed that night. "*Perhaps,*" he thought, "*there are worse things in life than being frozen.*" She may be frozen, but she was managing. In 50 years of anxiety and depression, she had found a way to survive, raise two girls, hold her marriage together, and now, on top of everything else, live with cancer. That was more than many could say. Her coping was clearly fragile, and perhaps she simply understood that choosing to "fight" her cancer would have overwhelmed her hard-won equilibrium.

"I have my struggles, but I'm still here and I'm still me." Maybe that, at the end of it all, was her message. She never gave the impression that she was expecting him to fix things. Maybe she just needed Dr. Parvinder to echo the message back to her: you are in tough straits, but you're a survivor and will find a way to cope.

"*Perhaps she is onto something,*" thought Dr. Parvinder as he closed his eyes. "*After all, freezing something is always the best way to preserve it.*"

4 A Falling Star

Barry Lavallee and Judith Belle Brown

"Doc, I am so fed up with feeling so tired all the time," said Sanjay as he slumped in the chair, while rubbing his eyes.

I had not seen 30-year-old Sanjay for some time. A healthy young man, he rarely came to the office, and when he did, it was normally for some minor problem. A wart. A flu shot. An ingrown toenail.

Sanjay's demeanor at this visit surprised me. His affect was flat and his frustration readily apparent. "Everything I try to do to remedy the situation just leaves me more tired. Like I played golf and met my friends for several games of tennis but nothing seems to help," he said with an exasperated tone in his voice. Sanjay went on to explain, "I have even given up fast foods and takeout, but even eating good wholesome meals is not helping." Sanjay strained to put on a smile about how good his life was despite his fatigue.

While I had seen Sanjay infrequently over the four years he had been my patient, I had come to know a few details about his life. After finishing high school, Sanjay had various jobs until he studied to become a realtor. He always saw himself as a high achiever. Sanjay enjoyed the challenge of "selling the most homes in a month" and often appeared in the gold category of his company, competing with national realtors. He felt pride in his accomplishments and being acclaimed as "a rising star" in the industry.

Thus as a realtor in a competitive market, Sanjay felt personal defeat at not being able to give 110% of himself all the time. He had worked hard to become "one of the best in the field" and now became anxious when the overwhelming sensation of tiredness engulfed him. Waking up each morning was a strain. "I am usually outgoing, love life and can work till I drop," Sanjay said wearily. He spoke with pride about carrying his beeper 24 hours a day. But Sanjay also wondered, "Maybe I should give the beeper up and take a night off. What do you think, Doc?" his eyes almost begging for permission.

When I asked if he had experienced anything like this before, Sanjay vaguely described an episode of "feeling down" several years ago. But just as I began to inquire further about the "episode," Sanjay's beeper sounded loudly. "Sorry Doc," he said quickly, "Gotta go. There's an offer coming in on my million-dollar listing. Guess you can't fix me today." Sanjay stood abruptly and as he exited the examining room, stated bluntly, "I'll be back."

It was several weeks before Sanjay returned and in interim I had been quietly concerned about the well-being of this normally gregarious young man. Something was wrong. When I entered the examination room my worst fears were realized. Sanjay had clearly lost more weight. He was unshaven and his eyes appeared bloodshot and puffy – almost as if he'd been crying. "I lost the million-dollar deal," he said mournfully, "and two other mega sales. What's happening to me, Doc? My life is falling apart big time." He sunk further into the chair. After a brief moment, Sanjay suddenly straightened up and, looking me in the eye, demanded, "You gotta give me something to fix me up and fast." I suspected there would be no quick fix and began to try and comprehend what was happening to Sanjay.

An inquiry of his illness experience revealed a six month history of fatigue and loss of interest in activities Sanjay had enjoyed in the past. He liked to go south to play golf with his friends and did so once a year. Sanjay played the stock market and was always on the lookout for a good investment. He talked about losing close to 80,000 dollars once and said it was part of the game. When asked if he had any close friends, Sanjay said, "I have many friends that I play golf and tennis with," but then sadly replied, "I don't have any close friends. Too busy." In addition, his girlfriend for the last two years had suddenly ended their relationship, claiming he loved his work more than her. Sanjay solemnly agreed, "I did love my work more than her. My work is my life." His eyes welled up with tears of shame.

Sanjay's appetite was down. "Geez Doc, I had to get all my pants altered, 'cause I've lost so much weight," Sanjay explained. He had periods when feelings of sadness flooded him. Fantasies of death came to him frequently, but Sanjay denied any fixed thoughts or plans to commit suicide. He worried more and more about how his work was affected and the potential loss of more clients. His sales had plummeted. Sanjay had overextended himself on his mortgage and a lavish automobile to impress his clients. His debts were rapidly accumulating.

Sanjay's despair permeated the room as his story unfolded. After some probing, Sanjay described a similar depressive episode following the breakup with his high school sweetheart when he was 22. His depression resolved after being treated with medication. He denied any other psychiatric illnesses such as mania or psychosis. Sanjay flatly denied alcohol or drug abuse. "Can't do that kind of stuff and work 18 hours a day. No way!" Sanjay was adamant in his response.

When asked about how he was feeling, Sanjay appeared guarded, as if not wanting to appear weak or inadequate. He struggled to preserve his persona of success. When asked to use more concrete words to describe his mood, Sanjay became tearful. These difficult moments were quickly coupled with tales of his many accomplishments. He clearly felt uncomfortable talking about the deeper issues affecting his life.

Over time, I learned that Sanjay was the eldest one of two siblings. His mother was alive and his father had died several years ago after a violent suicide. Sanjay had never forgiven his father and his anger ran deep. He did not spend much time with his brother and viewed him as a loser. "My brother has no ambition. You gotta have ambition to make it in this world," explained Sanjay – a man who was fighting desperately to maintain this long-held belief. His mother was needy and required much of Sanjay's attention, both financially and for many daily activities. It was wearing him down.

Whether Sanjay's current experience of depression was situational or hereditary appeared somewhat irrelevant. In order to help him, it was key to recognize this man's unique illness experience. In brief, Sanjay was terrified that his depression was eclipsing his life. He fought desperately to deny that his depression was his father's final legacy. His extremely successful career was in tatters. Sanjay often stated in desperation, "I am now a falling star." With many of his relationships on tenuous ground, he felt adrift as a worker, son and albeit "dumped" lover.

In time Sanjay came to realize that there would be no "quick fix". Working up to 18 hours per day and being reluctant to acknowledge the need for rest, Sanjay could only take small steps towards healing. During many moments when painful issues were discussed, Sanjay attempted to divert the conversation to more neutral territory. Eventually, Sanjay came to accept his depression. He agreed to try a course of medication. With careful monitoring, his mood stabilized and Sanjay overcame this episode of depression.

My therapeutic energy was directed at helping Sanjay achieve the ability to become more self-aware and to learn to prioritize and value his own needs. He became more comfortable in recognizing and accepting his needs as valid and worthy of attention. Sanjay continues to this day to "give the beeper up … sometimes for a whole weekend!" Perhaps as importantly, I came to value this patient's unique illness experience.

5 Living with a Chronic Illness

Sudha Koppula and Judith Belle Brown

As 33-year-old Olga Kesler slowly opened the door of her new family doctor's office, she paused abruptly, showered with anxiety. "*Will this doctor understand and help me?*" she fretted. Olga had moved here three months ago and it had taken her some time and effort to locate a family physician. By now her medications to control her Crohn's disease as prescribed by her gastroenterologist, located a thousand miles away, were running dangerously low. She was desperately in need of help. Over the last months, Olga had experienced several exacerbations of her Crohn's while traveling across the country on work-related assignments.

Suddenly, or so it seemed, Olga had met the man of her dreams: a man who shared a similar passion for the business of web design and expressed values and beliefs in concert with those of Olga. Within two months they were married. Together they decided to relocate their collective business ventures – and indeed their lives – to this new community.

As the door of the doctor's office closed, Olga trembled. "*So much has happened to me in the last few months,*" she silently reflected, "*what am I going to do? My Crohn's is getting worse and I can't let Damian know. He'll never understand.*" Olga fought back her tears as she approached the receptionist's desk.

Upon meeting Dr. Coulter, Olga recounted her story. Her primary medical concern was that her Crohn's disease had not been well-controlled in the past year. She had been previously followed by a gastroenterologist, but in the last year, as Olga crisscrossed the country, she had been forced to seek care from several emergency rooms for exacerbations of her Crohn's. Each time, the physicians in the various ERs had admonished Olga to stop work and receive appropriate treatment for her Crohn's. Yet she persisted on, driven by the need to excel in the new business she and her husband were launching nationwide. Olga knew she was her own worst enemy, but she couldn't help herself. "I want this project to succeed," was her ongoing mantra, and Olga would push her pain aside.

She had been diagnosed with Crohn's disease in her mid-20s. Since there was no family history of gastrointestinal problems, the diagnosis was a shock. Her previous family physician had suspected Crohn's disease after several weeks of weight loss, poor appetite, and bloody, diarrheal stools. With the help of a local gastroenterologist, Crohn's was diagnosed and was initially brought under control with medications alone. Olga had been symptom-free for almost five years until a year ago, when she began experiencing recurrent exacerbations, with no apparent trigger. The onset of her flare-ups coincided with the couple's decision to expand their business. "It was kind of bad timing," Olga explained. Olga did not understand why she had experienced so many severe Crohn's exacerbations in the past 12 months, as she felt she had been carefully monitoring her diet and strictly following her medication regimen.

Since her initial diagnosis, Olga had undergone a range of emotions. Initially, she was confused as to why this had happened to her when no one else in her family had experienced anything similar. Olga slowly came to terms with her diagnosis, which was made easier by the fact that her Crohn's initially came quickly under control easily with medical management.

When Dr. Coulter asked about her feelings about the exacerbation of her Crohn's, she clearly stated, "I feel very limited by it." More specifically, Olga explained, "I can't be far from a washroom when I have an exacerbation, I can't go out … sometimes I can't even eat. This past year has been very hard." With a warm smile on her face Olga added, "Sometimes it is hard to get to the washroom on a plane, especially during take-off and landing."

Olga explained to Dr. Coulter that she disliked having to take steroids because of the side effects of nausea and Cushingoid symptoms she suffered. She stoically described how her prior surgeries had been very difficult to endure. Previous procedures involved multiple colonoscopies, two prior bowel resections to remove the inflamed and damaged portions of her large intestine, and an appendectomy. Olga then stated one of her worst fears, "I hope I won't ever need a colostomy; that would be awful." However, Olga's greatest fear was the impact of her Crohn's disease on her ability to get pregnant and the implications this had on the future of her marriage.

A major dimension of Olga's illness experience was her role as a wife. She desperately wanted to maintain her sexual intimacy with her husband and of equal importance to fulfill their mutual desire to start a family. "Having children is a dream Damian and I both cherish," shared Olga, with tears filling her eyes. "I really worry about what will happen to us if I don't have a baby." Olga dabbed at her eyes with a tissue and took a deep breath. But Olga knew there were implications for whether or not she could conceive and then carry a pregnancy to term given the poor control of her Crohn's at the present time. Olga believed that if she could get her Crohn's disease under control, then she could reassure her husband about her health and the possibility of children in the future.

In the last few months, during the exacerbations, Olga described how her marriage to Damian had become more strained. "What does Damian know about Crohn's disease?" Dr. Coulter inquired gently.

"Oh, Damian is a smart man," Olga responded, quickly regaining her composure, "and he certainly understands what Crohn's is and how it affects me, at least theoretically," she added. Olga explained how Damian had known about her diagnosis prior to their marriage but had only been with her when she had been symptom-free. "So my flare-ups have been both a surprise and a worry for him," she said sadly, "and I know he is concerned about me. I think it frightens him to see me in such pain. And I recognize that I am a different person when I have a flare-up. I get quiet and pull away. It's not easy for Damian."

As a slight frown appeared on her face, Olga slowly continued. "But I know Damian struggles with the impact it has on our life together, in particular our sex life, which has been nil as of late." Olga's warm smile returned, "It is pretty hard to get pregnant if you don't have sex!" Just as quickly, she became serious again. "Damian now wonders if I will ever be healthy enough to get pregnant, and I wonder what will happen to our marriage if I can't!" Olga's tears returned.

Dr. Coulter carefully listened to Olga's experience of living with a chronic illness and acknowledged the many challenges she was currently facing. "How can I help you?" he inquired.

Olga's clearly articulated her expectations: she was in need of a family doctor who would help coordinate her care and refer her to a gastroenterologist for ongoing management of her Crohn's. She also expected her family doctor to listen to her concerns and advocate for her when required.

Olga understood that Crohn's disease is a chronic illness that can fluctuate between being controlled and exacerbating. But at this point in time, Olga was frustrated by her inability to get her Crohn's under control. Olga needed encouragement and hope that control could be regained and maintained. Olga also needed to be empowered to feel that she had a crucial role in the course of her illness.

Dr. Coulter addressed each of the dimensions of Olga's illness experience – her feelings and ideas about her Crohn's, how it was impacting her daily roles and responsibilities, and finally her expectations of her health care providers. By exploring not only her symptoms but also her unique experience of illness, he helped Olga regain control of her life. It also reminded Olga that she was not just a set of symptoms. In the future, the ongoing care by Dr. Coulter, her family physician, would be instrumental in helping Olga cope with the chronicity of her illness as well as its contextual implications as well.

"Thank you, Dr. Coulter," Olga said as she rose to leave the examination room. "In the last year I have felt like I was just a bundle of symptoms, but …" She paused for a moment as if searching for the right word or phrase. "But," she continued, clearing her throat, "today you made me feel, well this may sound silly, like a whole person. Thank you for that."

6 The Bear that Saved Her Life

Sudha Koppula and Judith Belle Brown

Claire Brice thought it was the perfect way to end a weekend away: her young son and daughter peacefully sleeping in the back seat of the van, her husband dozing next to her in the passenger seat. She relished the fact that she could play her soft music on the radio and have no one complain. It was dark, and the music helped her to focus.

On the right shoulder of the highway was something moving just ahead … the wind blowing some brush around, she thought, or an animal. Just as her headlights panned across the area, the answer became clear … the largest (and only) black bear she had ever encountered.

It was too late to avoid the bear. Had she been so stunned that she couldn't steer out of the way? Or was she too close in the first place? It didn't matter, she struck the bear, and as the van swerved and lurched after the impact, chaos penetrated the quiet night.

The kids awoke with a start. "What happened???" Her husband straightened himself up. "What did we hit?" As she braked and pulled onto the shoulder, she replied, "I hit a bear. I looked him right in the eye."

"Mom, I think he's dead," Claire's son replied. "Okay dear, just sit tight while your Dad and I step out and see about the bear," Claire responded.

Her husband rubbed his eyes. "I think it was a porcupine." Claire looked at him, surprised. "How would you know? You were asleep!" Claire's husband stepped down out of the van and looked at the newly-dented front fender, "That was one *big* porcupine."

The truck behind them slowed down and stopped along the shoulder as well. "You guys alright? That's one big bear you killed!"

"Told you it was a bear," Claire scoffed at her husband. She had been quite certain. "I looked him right in the eye."

The next morning Claire awoke with a grimace. "Ow, ow, ow!" Her husband was already awake and getting dressed. He saw her place her hand on her chest. "From the seatbelt, looks like. I have the same thing."

But he didn't have quite the same thing. As she pressed against her chest she became aware of something in addition to the soreness … a lump within her breast. She thought to herself, *"Huh. Never noticed that before. What is it? … A lump? Maybe I'll have my doctor check it out."* Claire felt it again: hard like a marble, only the one. *"I'll just have to put it out of my mind until I see her,"* she resolved.

Claire sat in an examining room at her doctor's office. "I hate these gowns," Claire thought. "Thirty-six years old and I still can't get used to them."

I knocked on the door and walked in. "Hi Claire! I hear you hit a bear?"

Claire just realized how incredible the story was, "Yep. I did. But the accident isn't the reason why I'm here ... I found this ..." Claire removed her gown and pointed to the area of her breast that she had been worried about.

"Mind if I examine it?" I asked.

"No, not at all," said Claire.

I palpated the area. It was the size of a small grape, round and hard. There was give to it like breast cysts usually have. The borders seemed regular, but I couldn't be sure. "Any others?" I asked. Claire shook her head to indicate no. "Perhaps I could examine both sides and under your arms, just to be thorough?" Claire was in agreement. She didn't want there to be any others.

"Well, looks like there's the one lump," I said. I was worried but didn't display my concern. "How about we arrange a few things – a mammogram, an ultrasound, and a biopsy."

Claire's mounting anxiety became apparent. "Do you think it's something serious?"

"Difficult to say, Claire. But there are some features of it that make me think we shouldn't just leave it alone. What do you think?"

Claire's eyes became wet with tears. "I'm scared. I wonder if it's breast cancer. I don't have a family history though ..." as her shaky voice trailed off.

I handed her a tissue and rested my hand on her shoulder, "How about we proceed as planned and we'll find out exactly what we're dealing with."

Claire sighed heavily, "I just want those tests to reassure me that it's nothing, just a cyst or something. My sister has those."

In closing I suggested: "Why don't we schedule a visit right after those investigations?" As Claire dried her tears, she nodded, thanked me and left.

The investigations occurred within the next week and the pathology report soon followed. I read it and thought to myself, *"DCIS – it did feel suspicious. I can't believe someone so young with no risk factors has breast cancer! I'd better have her come in right away."*

Claire was accompanied by her mom and sister at the next appointment. The three of them sat together holding hands. Claire dried away more tears. "They never call you in urgently for good news," she thought as she waited for what seemed like an eternity.

Another knock on the door, "Hi Claire," I said and then greeted her mom and sister. "I'm glad you're here too."

"So, what's the word?" Claire pointedly asked.

"Do you want just one word?" I replied.

Claire quickly responded, "Just the bottom line, please, doctor."

Slowly I said: "Okay Claire… It's cancer."

There were more tears, this time from Claire as well as her mother and sister. I slowly took a seat and waited. A jumble of thoughts filled my mind beyond the clinical significance of this encounter. Such a young patient, no family history, young children … doesn't seem fair … not that it's fair for anyone who has cancer, but somehow more unfair in this situation. I waited and held Claire's hand.

"I guess I knew it … What's next, doctor?" Claire dried her tears and looked stoic.

I explained the referrals, tests and potential interventions, then paused and asked, "Do you have any questions or anything you want to talk about?"

Claire quickly responded, "No … thanks for offering though. I think I already knew … I just really want to get rid of it."

Within two weeks, Claire was seen by a surgeon. "Did you really hit a bear?" Her surgeon asked, surprised. He arranged for a lumpectomy and a speedy referral to the cancer center. The surgery was performed without any complications, and the lymph nodes were negative. Even so, Claire was offered chemotherapy and radiation by the cancer center because of her young age. "I'll do everything to get rid of this cancer," she told them. Her medical and radiation oncologists asked the same question, "Did you really hit a bear?" And she replied to them all. "Yes, I hit a bear."

Weeks of nausea, fever, poor appetite and general malaise followed. I received update after update from the cancer center that I read and filed in her chart. I reflected, "*Looks like she's having a tough time. I wonder if I should call her.*" I did and left a message to come in when Claire felt she was able. I wondered if it might be helpful to reflect on this experience together.

Claire came for a follow-up appointment with the expressed intent of ensuring I was up-to-date on everything that had happened. "I'm doing fine, doctor," she reassured me. "Radiation is planned. I can't wait to get on with that and have this all over. Chemo is a nightmare … but I'm getting used to it. What a terrible thing to say, don't you think? Even the nausea isn't bad anymore because I can anticipate when that's going to happen, and I know how to manage it, so it's not that bad. They tell me my hair will grow back." She rubbed her fuzzy bald head and laughed.

I didn't say much, but welcomed learning about Claire's experiences. I was relieved to hear that she was coping well. Claire looked very different from her usual self, but her resolve was very evident. She drew much strength from her family. Even her two young children had been encouraging to her. She was proud of all of them and felt lucky for the wonderful people in her life who were helping her through this journey.

As the visit came to a close, I reflected, "I'm so happy to hear you have so much support to help you through it."

"Thanks … You remember how you asked me if I really hit that bear?" said Claire.

"Yes, I do. It was a remarkable story!" I exclaimed.

"Well, everyone I met in the hospital, nurses, doctors, nutritionists, everyone keeps asking me the same question! Did you know that my son's nickname has been 'Bear' ever since he was born?" asked Claire.

"Really? That's interesting …" I said.

Claire continued, "And everyone keeps giving me bear angel figurines as presents now! They are thankful for that bear. Had it not been for him …" Claire's voice trailed away.

"…we never would have known about that lump," as I completed her thought.

"I looked him right in the eye. You know, black bears usually don't come out at night like that," said Claire softly.

"Maybe he was there for a reason."

"Yes", reflected Claire, "It appears that way."

Smiling, I said "Good thing for that bear."

"A very good thing …" Claire responded, also smiling.

7 Conquering Pain and Fear

Dori Seccareccia and Judith Belle Brown

"I can't take it anymore, I just don't want to go on with this much pain, I'd rather be dead," Dianne said through clenched teeth, her face contorted in pain. Dianne had been admitted to the palliative care unit for management of intractable left leg pain secondary to an inoperable chondrosarcoma in her pelvis.

Dianne had been diagnosed during the birth by C-section of her second son, Nicholas. It was a time of joy and sorrow. She underwent surgery and chemotherapy. For a year she felt well and renewed as a mother and wife. Then the tumor recurred and was deemed inoperable. Dianne did not want further chemotherapy because of how sick she had felt during her previous treatments, and thus far had put a hold on radiation therapy. On this occasion she had been admitted to hospital to investigate a new onset of increased leg swelling and pain. Once it was determined that it was not due to a venous thrombosis, Dianne was transferred to the palliative care unit for pain control. Her one and only goal when she arrived on the unit was, "You have to make the pain STOP!"

When Dianne described her experience of having cancer, two central themes emerged: fear and guilt. Dianne's fears had been escalating as the reality of her situation became readily apparent. When first diagnosed, Dianne refused to believe that she would not be completely cured. But the growing tumor in her pelvis and the increasing pain were constant reminders of her unrelenting disease and her own mortality. Dianne openly spoke of the fear of the pain persisting and escalating, and of dying in pain. Without restraint, she also vented her anger about her horrific pain, "Can't you get rid of this GD pain? What if it's worse tomorrow? What if the medicine you are trying works and then stops working? Why can't you just cut the whole leg off and get rid of the cancer?" Her anguish filled the room. Dianne's expectations were abundantly clear.

Dianne did not remember what it felt like not to be in pain and to not be tired. While Dianne was terrified by her pain, she also had remarkable insight into how her fear intensified her pain, thus making it harder to control. Pain symbolized disease to her, and the more pain, the more disease – and the more disease, the closer she was to dying. But for Dianne, something was out of order in the universe when she, a 31-year-old mother of two, was dying. She had lost her ability to be the kind of mother she wanted to be, the kind of wife she wanted to be, and the kind of woman she wanted to be.

Dianne had two sons, Wayne, age six, and Nicholas, who was just turning three. She adored their energy, exuberance, and the warmth of their loving embraces. But her guilt about not being at home and being able to care for them was overwhelming. So was her guilt that she would soon die and leave them motherless. Dianne's guilt was compounded by the fact that when she was in such terrible pain, she often lost her temper with her young sons when they came to visit her in hospital. Being in constant pain prevented her from being the positive and energetic mom she expected to be. Her guilt and remorse was blatant when Dianne stated, "I hate myself, but I can't help losing it when my leg hurts so much and they're jumping all over me and not listening." Her guilt also surfaced when she would become angry with her husband, George, for not being able to make her feel better. Flooded with emotion, Dianne exclaimed, "He's my best friend and I treat him like garbage!" When her family left, Dianne would lie in her hospital bed wracked by guilt and her uncontrollable sobs.

Dianne had been married to George for 10 years. Having started their relationship as high school sweethearts, Dianne considered George the most important source of support in her life. "I know that George would sell the house and steal money to buy me a cure if there was one," she said proudly. He had always accompanied Dianne to all of her appointments and multiple cancer treatments in the past. Now he was torn between remaining vigilant at his wife's bedside and caring for their two young boys.

At the beginning, George also believed that Dianne would be fully cured, but lately he had been talking more about how he would cope when she died. "I'm not stupid," he said plainly, "I can see the writing on the wall. I just want her to be comfortable and be with us as long as possible, but I don't want her to be at home and in pain." George paused, his profound grief almost preventing him from carrying on, "It's too hard on everyone."

When Dianne was first diagnosed, she required a lot of help. People were generally there for her. When she was in remission, she was fairly independent. When Dianne became ill again, her supports were limited. "The worse I become, the more I find out who my real friends are, and they are great," she stated stoically. "I am a strong person. I am not a quitter, but this pain is wearing me down," Dianne expressed emphatically.

She had some regrets but did not ruminate about them. "What's the point in dwelling on the past?" she reflected. "I must focus on the future, perhaps not mine, but that of my family," she commented with clear resolve. When Dianne was not in pain she worked diligently on organizing her sons' and husband's lives for when she was not there. Dianne had been forced to alter the entire blueprint she had designed for her future. The deep remorse in her voice was evident when Dianne said, "I won't be able to watch the kids grow up and have their own lives." Sadly she continued on, "All the dreams George and I had for the future are gone."

Her ability to live her life as she wanted was shattered because of a life-limiting illness. The independence and control she cherished had been suddenly stripped away because of her illness. Dianne explained, "I don't care who you are or what you've been through, there is no way you can understand how much pain I'm having and what it's like being stuck in this hospital bed and not in your own home, cut off from your family".

As clinicians, it is perhaps easy to talk about focusing on hope, but when you must relinquish all your life-long dreams, it can be overwhelming. And what makes it more overwhelming is having to do it while in pain. Pain wears you down and does not allow you to be who you really are. Having faced this degree of pain will certainly leave one with an enormous fear of the pain persisting, and if it ever resolves, that it will return. Dianne certainly exhibited these fears. Dianne's pain clearly had a large physical component, but also emotional, social and spiritual aspects. When her left leg would begin to ache, Dianne would worry that the cancer was growing, and she would ask herself the basic existential question "why me?"

8 Facing an Incurable Condition

Sharon Nur Hatcher and Judith Belle Brown

Mrs. Suzzette Lachine was a 68-year-old woman who presented with progressive shortness of breath over the last year that had been diagnosed as asthma. However, her inhalers were not helping, and she was increasingly concerned about her stamina. She had come to be my patient at the request of her daughter, who was already a patient of the practice. Her daughter hoped I could discover what was truly ailing her mother.

Mrs. Lachine's illness experience revolved around the fear of the loss of autonomy and her capacity to care for her husband, who had recently been diagnosed with Alzheimer's disease. She was already grieving the loss of the life she had with her husband of 50 years. Mrs. Lachine was sad and resistant to the idea of his eventual placement in a nursing home. At this point, Mrs. Lachine had no outside help in the home. But as she explained, "I always worry about the safety of my husband when I must leave the house to run errands." She had little distress about her own health, which had always been good in the past. Except for now. "I just have this inner feeling that something more serious is amiss," she said with worry in her voice. "I have felt like my health has been going downhill in the last six months and no one is taking my concerns seriously." Mrs. Lachine wanted some answers, in the hope of getting a clearer diagnosis.

Besides her history of shortness of breath and fatigue, Mrs. Lachine had few other symptoms. Her difficulty breathing manifested itself as soon as she started to walk, and she had to pause frequently in order to recover. She had no chest pain, no cough, no nocturnal symptoms, and no fever. Her appetite had decreased somewhat and she had lost some weight – "perhaps five pounds," she reported. Other than that, she had been in remarkably good health prior to the onset of these symptoms.

I examined Mrs. Lachine on several recurring visits. She was a petite woman, 95 pounds and barely five feet tall. Her salt-and-pepper curls framed her smiling face. Surprisingly, auscultation of her lungs and heart was not helpful: a few non-specific basilar rales. Examination of her abdomen revealed no significant findings. There was no lymphadenopathy. It was at the end of one visit that I glanced at her hands: there had been a change, even in the short time I had been following her. They were pale with red telangiectasias, and the skin on her fingers was atrophied and tight. Upon further questioning, she said she was having trouble manipulating objects and even had a small persistent ulcer on her finger.

Blood work was not helpful, except for assisting in diagnosing an inflammatory type of anemia. A chest X-ray was essentially normal. I referred her to the pulmonary specialist for a bronchoscopy and to the dermatologist, who both confirmed what I was suspecting: Mrs. Lachine had systemic scleroderma.

Mrs. Lachine was a gentle and unassuming person. She had not benefitted from much education and had devoted her life to raising five daughters and taking care of her family. Despite facing multiple hardships, Mrs. Lachine never complained. On the contrary, she would often state in a matter-of-fact tone, "I have had a good life. I have no complaints. Indeed I have been blessed." Her daughters adored her but were faced with the demands of their own families and careers. As Mrs. Lachine explained quite plainly, "They all lead busy lives – I don't want to bother them." Her daughters were increasingly sad and distressed about this incurable disease that their mother didn't "deserve." Instead, she certainly deserved peace and a well-earned rest in her latter years. However, Mrs. Lachine faced her diagnosis with resignation. She minimized her impairment and pain. Mrs. Lachine had always been proudly independent and resilient. "I have never asked anything of anyone," she expressed firmly. But all of a sudden, in a short period of time, she was losing everything: her husband, her house, her life.

The life cycle issue at the forefront of Mrs. Lachine's preoccupation was the care of her deteriorating husband. Even with increasing help at home, her own health problems now prevented her from caring for him. This was very difficult for her to accept - at times her grief and guilt were paralyzing. She felt that his upcoming admission to a long-term care facility would cause him great distress. "He will never be able to overcome this move," Mrs. Lachine said with a deep sadness. They had lived happily together in their home for many years, and the sudden changes were overwhelming. At the same time, Mrs. Lachine demonstrated characteristic fortitude and courage. "C'est la vie," she would sigh.

There was a special trust that Mrs. Lachine and her family had invested in me, given that I had made the diagnosis that remained elusive for many months. But I knew I was just present at the right time when the signs of the disease became more evident. I tried to use this trust to help Mrs. Lachine express her emotions about the upsetting difficulties she was experiencing and assist her in the grieving process. As winter set in and Mrs. Lachine's health deteriorated, her care became essentially palliative. The care provided rapidly transitioned from managing her chronic disease to providing palliative care with the accompanying end-of-life decisions and grief process.

Mrs. Lachine's story raises many issues facing an elderly person encountering an incurable condition. Now a patient, she was also a caregiver of a husband with Alzheimer's disease, which in itself carries a tremendous load of grief and major adaptation. While adapting to a loss of autonomy and function, the illness also had repercussions for all members of the family. The adult children of the patient were, in a very short span of time, required to dramatically increase the care and support for their parents as well as accept help from previously known community resources. As their family physician, I was able to identify and address the many physical, emotional, social and spiritual needs of my patient and her family. The major challenge lay in the fact that initially all these issues were not readily apparent. A patient-centered approach was critical to the process of assessment and problem identification, long before treatment and management could even be discussed.

This case also illustrates the process by which a primary care physician uses a clinical method to assess and investigate undifferentiated presenting symptoms. At first, common hypotheses are formed and verified. If these do not fit, it is often follow-up over a period of time, coupled with keen observation and attentiveness, that will lead to a clearer understanding and definition of the patient's problems. These include not only a physical disease process, which in this case happened to be irreversible, but also the impact of that disease on the patient's function, person and family.

In conclusion, like many chronic and incurable diseases, management of Mrs. Lachine's condition did not involve major specialist care, but rather mobilizing community resources for supportive palliative care. No one who cared for Mrs. Lachine had ever treated a patient with scleroderma before. This fact was largely irrelevant to her quality of care, which depended more on an attentive sensitivity to her unique condition and to her illness experience, as well as on creative solutions in order to provide Mrs. Lachine and her family optimal comfort.

9 Clearing the Path

Jana Malhotra and Judith Belle Brown

"I need a note for more time off work," Carmen stated bluntly. Her affect was flat and her mood uncharacteristically low.

Dr. Alexander, Carmen's family physician, was somewhat surprised by the shroud of helplessness that appeared to envelope this usually outspoken 19 year old. Dr. Alexander knew that Carmen's life had not been easy. Her parents divorced when Carmen was 12, and as an only child she became the caretaker of her alcoholic mother. That role ceased abruptly when Carmen's mother was incarcerated for impaired driving and leaving the scene of an accident. Child protection services placed 13-year-old Carmen in foster care. She ran away on multiple occasions. At the age of 15, Carmen was diagnosed with depression, and then at age 16 she became pregnant and quit school. The baby's father, unwilling to assume the responsibilities of parenthood, abandoned Carmen upon learning that she was pregnant.

All these events had transpired prior to Dr. Alexander becoming Carmen's family physician. He had first met her early in her pregnancy, had been present at Jordan's birth, and had seen them both regularly in the clinic for well-baby checks over the last 18 months. In spite of the many challenges in her short life, Dr. Alexander had high regard for Carmen's spunk and determination.

Carmen had recently moved out of supportive housing and rented a small, one-bedroom apartment. She had found a part-time job at a neighborhood convenience store and managed to secure subsidized daycare for Jordan while she was at work. The move had been a struggle for Carmen, as she was now responsible for both herself and her 18-month-old son. But she was coping and proud of the life she was building for the two of them. The chaos of her past appeared to be receding.

Then the car accident happened. It occurred while Carmen was a passenger in her boyfriend's car, which was rear ended while stopped at a red light. Carmen suffered a Colles' fracture of her left wrist when she braced her hand on the dashboard as the vehicle slammed into the intersection, striking another car. No one else had been injured, but nonetheless the accident had been a distressing event for Carmen. Although she was right-handed, it was still very difficult for her to care for her son Jordan, especially since he was becoming such a busy toddler. Carmen's guilt about not being able to look after her son as best she could was most evident. Carmen was barely coping.

Through a veil of tears Carmen explained, "I just feel so overwhelmed and exhausted. I don't feel like I am being a good enough mother to little Jordan, and I am very worried about my finances because of being off work. I just feel so helpless right now. I can't figure out what to do," she said with dismay. Carmen continued on, explaining how she was feeling under tremendous pressure to quickly return to work, as her job was in jeopardy. "But how can I go back to work? I stock shelves and work the cash register," Carmen gulped for air as if suffocating under the weight of her responsibilities. "I can hardly care for me and Jordan, let alone work at the store. Oh man, what am I going to do, I can't lose this job!"

In addition, Carmen was also concerned about her relationship with her new boyfriend, Mauricio. Carmen and Mauricio had started fighting since the accident, and the tension between them was escalating. He couldn't comprehend why an injury to her non-dominant hand should cause her so much difficulty. In contrast, Carmen felt Mauricio could be more supportive and understanding. Cautiously she stated, "I thought that he might move in with us so he could help me out with Jordan while I have my cast on, even though Jordan isn't his baby. The accident was his fault, after all!" The growing discord in her relationship with Mauricio was obviously causing Carmen distress. "What is it with me and guys?" she asked with a hint of anger in her voice. "Just when I think I have finally met 'Mr. Right,' he turns out to be a jerk!" she snorted. Carmen's voice quickly softened. "No, that's not fair, I know Mauricio loves me and Jordan. The accident was hard on him too. But we gotta get it together and stop fighting!" Carmen's tears returned, and under the stress, her hopelessness resurfaced. This young woman's life was in disarray once again.

Generally, Carmen was a healthy young woman, with no medical problems apart from a previous history of depression when she was 15. For over two years her mood had been stable, and she was not currently on any medication. Carmen did not have any significant pain or discomfort from her distal radius fracture. Her cast was in good condition, she had normal capillary refill and normal power and range of motion in her fingers on the right hand.

But something was not right in Carmen's world. In addition to her Colles' fracture, Carmen was now complaining of general fatigue, a depressed mood and difficulty sleeping. "I am just very tired. It's not like how I felt after Jordan was born. This is different." Carmen explained in a weary tone, "Maybe I'm just wrung out from all the worry." Her appetite was normal and her weight stable. Carmen denied any suicidal or homicidal ideation, nor was she having hallucinations.

Briefly, Carmen's mood brightened as she exclaimed, "I've got every-thing to live for, Jordan is the light of my life!" Her face darkened again. "Oh geez, am I getting depressed again? This can't be happening!" Carmen's body shuddered as the shroud of helplessness descended again.

Carmen had developed a strong and trusting relationship with her family physician and expected Dr. Alexander to help her deal with her concerns. She came to the office frequently, and was usually quite adamant about what she expected from the encounter. But on this occasion Dr. Alexander noted how Carmen appeared unclear about what she wanted or needed. Knowing Carmen's previous history allowed Dr. Alexander to understand that his patient was not her usual self during this visit. While Carmen's life was crisis-ridden, she had never appeared this helpless before. Carmen was clearly suffering from her overwhelming situation.

As Dr. Alexander explored Carmen's illness experience, he silently reflected, "Carmen is having difficulty coping with this new change in her physical health. I wonder, has this precipitated a depressive episode? While this is common in patients suffering from severe medical conditions such as cancer, it is unusual for patients with more minor physical ailments."

While listening to Carmen's story, Dr. Alexander found himself strug-gling with the identification of an accurate diagnosis. Was Carmen suffering from an adjustment disorder or depression? By delving into Carmen's expe-rience of illness and her current difficulties, it was evident that she required a significant amount of support and reassurance. The actual label did not matter as much as understanding her illness experience and deciding on the most appropriate treatment plan.

Given Carmen's current symptoms, which had been ongoing for a few weeks, and her previous history of depression, together the patient and doctor agreed to start her on a low-dose antidepressant. Although initially hesitant, Carmen acknowledged how medication had helped her battle depression in the past. Carmen readily agreed to attend a support group at the local mental health center. Because of the relationship bond Carmen had established with Dr. Alexander, she was more than willing to continue having individual visits with him on a weekly basis until she regained some mastery over her life situation. "Maybe Mauricio might even come to a few sessions," she asked hopefully.

"He is more than welcome," responded Dr. Alexander with encouragement.

At the conclusion of the visit, Carmen was relieved. "So there is some-thing more wrong with me and we can fix it – right?" she asked hopefully. Carmen knew she would have the support to help her deal with her current difficulties. As Carmen left the office, Dr. Alexander handed her a note for her workplace, stating she was not able to return to work at this point in time. "Thanks Dr. A!" she said, grasping the note in her hand, "You're a lifesaver!" Carmen stood smiling in the doorway.

"No, no, Carmen. You're in charge of your life. I'm just helping you along the way, trying to clear the path a bit," responded Dr. Alexander as the dark cloud around them lifted.

10 A Ray of Hope

Nusrat Jamil and Judith Belle Brown

Dr. Horowitz had struggled in his care of Lilly Chui during the first 10 years of their relationship. She dismissed his recommendations regarding the treatment of her uncontrolled hypertension, hypercholesterolemia and type 2 diabetes. Lilly wanted to avoid "pills" and was adamant that "I just want to do it more naturally." Yet her lifestyle changes were minimal, and other than light housework Lilly remained quite sedentary. But Lilly was a ticking time bomb. Concurrent with her own health problems, Lilly's family history was ominous – both of her parents had suffered debilitating strokes secondary to hypercholesterolemia. Her two elderly brothers had died of pancreatic cancer within six months of each other.

Turning 65 had been a watershed for Lilly. Much to Dr. Horowitz's amazement, Lilly decided to actively take control of her health. Lilly started walking a little over a mile a day when the weather was fair, and when it became inclement, she took to her treadmill with a vengeance. She attended classes at the Diabetic Education Center, determined to begin cooking healthy meals for her and her husband, Wang.

When Lilly had initially reported her sudden lifestyle changes to improve her health and reduce her risk factors, Dr. Horowitz had been skeptical. What caused this sudden change in Lilly at age 65? He wondered: had it been the sudden death of her two brothers in their early 70s? The increasing care required by her husband, who was 10 years her senior? The birth of her first grandchild? Or all of the above? He might never really know what had motivated Lilly to take charge of her health. What did matter was that Lilly had sustained these lifestyle changes now for five years. Dr. Horowitz was both pleased and impressed.

Now Lilly was complaining of swelling, pain and a burning sensation in her left hand, wrist and forearm for the last two weeks. Lilly had suffered a Colles' fracture 12 weeks ago secondary to a fall on her outstretched hand while venturing outside for a walk on a less-than-perfect day. She presented to the emergency room, and a temporary cast was put on her forearm. Lilly was later seen in the cast clinic, and a full cast was placed on her forearm for six weeks. The cast had been removed two weeks ago, and since then Lilly had been experiencing severe pain in her left hand, wrist and forearm. In her mind, she had almost recovered from her recent left Colles' fracture, but now she had this unrelenting pain. The pain was compromising her ability to sleep or do anything with her left hand. Lilly was very worried about this new onset of pain. "What's causing this?" she asked, her face red and blotchy from crying.

Lilly had reached a stage in her life where she had taken control of her health. She felt proud of her newfound lease on life – or so she thought. These new symptoms represented a loss of control over her health issues despite her best efforts. "I just feel so helpless," Lilly said through her tears. "I worked very hard to take charge of my health and now this happens!" Dr. Horowitz handed Lilly another tissue and continued to listen. "I've been crying nonstop and that's just not like me – I have always been a fighter," she said as the tears flowed down her cheeks, "but right now I can't fight these feelings of sadness." Lilly was unable to differentiate whether the crying spells and loss of sleep were due to the severity of her pain or a result of her feelings of helplessness and present loss of control over her health.

The pain was severely limiting Lilly's ability to fulfill her day to day role as a homemaker. Her husband, Wang, depended on Lilly for many of his daily needs, both physical and emotional. Lilly was exhausted by her lack of sleep for the last two weeks. This was largely because of the pain, compounded by the anxiety and worry about her health. Lilly had reluctantly tried Tylenol, which had not been of much help to her.

Lilly's expectations of this visit were very clear to Dr. Horowitz as she rapidly stated, "What's wrong with my arm? Why has the fracture not healed? It has been three months! Why am I having so much pain now?" Lilly paused, caught her breath, and through her multiple tears begged, "Please Dr. Horowitz, I need to sleep and to manage at home so I can take care of Wang – and me too!"

Gently, Dr. Horowitz tried to reassure Lilly that he would do whatever he could to understand her problem and help her regain control of her health. "Lilly, I know you have worked very hard to get healthy," he said. "You have made some amazing changes in your life, and the improvement in your health has been awesome." Lilly smiled with his praise. Dr. Horowitz continued, "So Lilly, this current situation is very distressing and worrisome. I know you are frightened." His words appeared to temper Lilly's sense of desperation.

Dr. Horowitz acknowledged the severity of her pain, and suggested that she could be suffering from complex regional pain syndrome type 1 (CRPS). He explained to her that CRPS is a disease in which the nervous system malfunctions in a way that causes the pain to escalate even the original injury has healed. The symptoms of sadness Lilly was feeling commonly accompanied the diagnosis. Lilly recognized she was feeling sad and anxious but was not sure whether this was due to her pain and/or her feelings of deep sadness about not being able to engage in her daily activities of healthy living. Also, the fear of the unknown was frightening her. Lilly also expressed grief over the loss of control of her health despite her best efforts in the last five years. She had worked so hard.

Lilly usually refused medications, but in this new situation she willingly agreed to treat the pain, and then slowly taper the medication as the symptoms subsided. A subsequent X-ray of her wrist showed evidence of a healed Colles' fracture. A bone scan confirmed radiological evidence consistent with the diagnosis of CRPS. Dr. Horowitz offered Lilly a trial of prednisone but also cautioned that her blood sugar levels might be difficult to control while she was taking steroids. Lilly refused the prednisone, as Dr. Horowitz had expected. However, patient and doctor did agree on a plan that included controlling her pain with medications and aggressive physiotherapy, without compromising her diabetic control, which Lilly had worked so diligently to attain.

CRPS is an important diagnosis to make, as the unrelenting pain can cause many patients much physical and emotional misery – as it did for Lilly. Having a diagnosis helped Lilly feel less devastated by her illness experience. It gave her a ray of hope.

COMPONENT II

Understanding the Whole Person

Judith Belle Brown, W. Wayne Weston and Thomas R. Freeman

We all face the many challenges and demands presented at each stage of human development. The ascendancy to independence in adolescence, the creation of intimate partnerships in adulthood, the realignment of roles and tasks that transpire in the senior years are all examples of expected life-cycle changes. How we traverse each stage will be influenced by prior life experience. For many individuals, the successful achievement of the tasks and expectations of each developmental phase steers them through life relatively unscathed. But for others, each ensuing life phase may be marred by past failures and previous losses. For them, life's challenges are experienced as overwhelming and often unachievable.

The second component of the patient-centered clinical method is the integration of the concepts of health, disease and illness with an understanding of the whole person, including an awareness of the patient's position in the life cycle and his or her life context. The patient's position in the life cycle takes into consideration the individual's own personality development, whereas the patient's context includes both proximal, i.e. familial, and distal, i.e. cultural, contexts.

THE PERSON: INDIVIDUAL DEVELOPMENT

Understanding patients' perceptions of health, disease(s) and unique illness experience is only one aspect of their personhood. They are children, partners, parents, aunts and uncles, friends and colleagues who have a past, a present and a future. The motives, attachments, ideals, and expectations that shape their personality evolve as they ascend each developmental phase.

Healthy individual development is reflected by a solid sense of self, positive self-esteem, and a position of independence and autonomy, coupled with the capacity for connectedness and intimacy (Erikson, 1950, 1982; Jordan, Kaplan and Miller, *et al*. 1991; Bowlby 1973; Bowlby 1982; Broderick and Blewitt 2010; Guest 2007; Harris 2011; Santrock 2007; Schriver 2004). Their lives are greatly influenced by each developmental phase, which may be isolated and lonely, e.g. for a homeless woman, or vast and complex, e.g. for a middle-aged man recently diagnosed with diabetes and facing the multiple responsibilities of husband, father, son and worker. Thus their position in the life cycle, the tasks they assume, and the roles they ascribe to, will influence the care they seek.

Understanding the patient's current stage of development and the relevant developmental tasks that need to be accomplished can assist doctors in several ways. First, knowledge of the predictable tasks of each life stage that occur in individual development helps the physician recognize the patient's problems as more than isolated, episodic phenomena. Also, being aware of prior losses or developmental crises assists the doctor to identify vulnerable junctures in the patient's life. For example, knowing that a patient has minimal family interaction or limited social supports alerts the physician to an individual at risk. Second, it can increase the doctor's sensitivity to the multiple factors that influence the patient's problems and broaden awareness of the impact of the patient's life history. Third, an understanding of the whole person enhances the physician's interaction with the patient and may be particularly helpful when signs or symptoms do not point to a clearly defined disease process or when the patient's response to an illness appears exaggerated or out of character. On these occasions, it is often helpful to explore how the patient is dealing with the common issues related to his or her stage in the life cycle. Finally, understanding the whole person may also expand the doctor's level of comfort with caring as well as curing.

CONTEXT: PROXIMAL AND DISTAL FACTORS

Context is defined by those factors that are proximal and those that are distal to the patient. Proximal factors correspond most closely to with those that are immediate and specific to the patient, whereas distal factors are more closely aligned with the general categories and are common to groups of people living in the same locale. The boundaries between the proximal and distal factors are to a great extent artificial, as the interaction between them is both dynamic and bidirectional.

Proximal factors include: family, financial security, education, employment, leisure and social support. Distal factors include: culture, community, economics, the health care system, socio-historical issues, geography, the media and ecosystem health.

Therefore, both proximal and distal contexts are composed of multiple factors that impact the individual's experience of health, disease and the illness experience. These contexts also influence and shape individual development. Two examples are discussed below: for the proximal context, the role of the family is examined, with culture serving as the example of a distal factor in context.

PROXIMAL FACTOR: THE FAMILY

People linked by blood, marriage or close emotional attachment constitute a family. The field of family systems theory sees the family as a mutually interacting system functioning as an emotional unit. As Scarf (1995, p. xxii) so eloquently states: the family unit can be viewed as "... a great emotional foundry, the passion-filled forge in which our deepest realities – our sense of who we are as persons, and of the world around us – first begins to form and take shape. It is within the enclave of the early family that we learn those patterns of being, both of a healthy and a pathological nature, which will gradually be assimilated into, and becoming a fundamental part of, our own inner experience."

Illness is a powerful agent of change. The burden of illness, either acute or chronic, may cause severe disruption even to the most functional family system by altering how family members relate (Ransom 1993; Rolland 1989; Harris 2011; Gorman 2011; Sawicki 2011). It may ultimately impede their ability to overcome the ramifications of the illness experience (McDaniel, Campbell and Seaburn 1990; Gorman 2011). Major changes in routine, such as care of a child with a life-limiting diagnosis or care of an elderly parent, may demand a change in the family role structure and task allocation.

The family disequilibrium resulting from illness also can alter the established rules and expectations of the family members and transform their methods of communication. The changes imposed on families by illness are almost limitless and accompanied by a host of feelings, both negative and positive: loss, fear, anger, resignation, anxiety, sadness, resentment, dependency, as well as a sense of privilege for the opportunity of giving and caring.

How families have coped previously will influence how they experience the impact of the illness on their family roles, rules, patterns of communication and structures. Therefore, in understanding the impact of the illness on the family, some key questions can guide the doctor's inquiry. At what stage is the family in its life cycle, e.g. starting a family, retirement? Where is each member in the life cycle, e.g. adolescence, middle age? What are the developmental tasks for each individual and for the family as a whole? How does the illness affect the achievement of these multiple tasks? What kinds of illnesses has the family experienced? What kinds of support have they mobilized in the past to help them cope with illness? Is there currently an established support network? How has the family dealt with illness in the past? Have they responded with functional or dysfunctional patterns of behavior? For example, has the family demonstrated potential maladaptive responses, such as rejection of the sick person, or overprotection that stifles responsibility for self-care? It is often helpful for clinicians to ask patients who they seek assistance from when a family member is ill.

These latter questions are important because they elicit how families may contribute to or perpetuate illness behavior in their members. The family may represent a safe refuge for the ill person or, conversely, may aggravate the illness through maladaptive responses.

DISTAL FACTOR: CULTURE

Culture has a profound impact on how patients experience health care. The way patients conceptualize and interpret their illness is strongly determined by cultural affiliation. Cultural norms and values influence how patients view health and disease, experience illness, seek care and accept medical interventions (Kleinman, Eisenberg and Good 1978; Helman 2007).

There are several cultural features to consider for each of the five aspects (health, disease, illness, person and context) of the whole person in this model. Perceptions of health are dictated by culture, and although disease is explained by the conventional medical model, it is not immune to the influence of culture. The conventional medical model and the scientific method are both products of Western culture. Hence, our cultural "filters" affect how we, as clinicians, understand and manage diseases (Juckett 2005). Just as the approaches to medical practice differ, the venues employed by patients in meeting their health care needs also vary. In North America, patient autonomy trumps other values such as beneficence, whereas other cultures place more value on beneficence. These different cultural values have a major influence on the patient-physician relationship and the approach to finding common ground about management decisions (Searight and Gafford 2005).

Patients' experience of illness will be profoundly influenced by cultural beliefs about "appropriate" illness behavior and models of care. What counts as a symptom of illness and when to consult family members, lay practitioners, healers or traditional health care professionals are all prescribed by culture (Juckett 2005).

Culture has a fundamental effect on the psychological development of the person. A move from one culture to another involves major upheaval and loss, which may have serious effects on self-esteem (Sawicki 2011; Pottie *et al.* 2005). Such a transition may be compounded by the trauma of torture and the humiliation of refugee status (Pottie *et al.* 2005). Language barriers make it even more difficult to articulate needs and to receive support.

There are different cultural responses to transitions in the family life cycle such as pregnancy, labor, childbirth and care of the elderly and dying (Searight and Gafford 2005). Cultural differences in family roles and rules may come into conflict with the expectations of the doctor. For example, some cultural groups actively protect terminally ill family members from information about the severity of their condition, making end-of-life decision-making a challenge (Searight and Gafford 2005).

What strategies can the doctor use to learn more about the patient's culture? It is the doctor's responsibility to attempt to bridge the cultural gap by becoming as familiar as possible with the patient's cultural traditions and beliefs (Juckett 2005; Rosenberg *et al.* 2007). For example, it may be useful to explain to patients that it would help the doctor, in caring for them, to know more about the patient and his or her home situation, and the individual's native country. Doctors can point out that they are not experts in other cultures and that they need patients' help to understand them better. This is where it is important to distinguish between cultural humility and cultural competence (Trevalon and Murray-Garcia 1998). A doctor might ask for tolerance if he says or does something that would be inappropriate in the patient's homeland, and he may encourage the patient to inform him so that he does not repeat the same mistake. This disclosure may be difficult for some patients if they are accustomed to viewing doctors as authorities, or if their life experiences have socialized them to respond to authority figures with deference, submissiveness or fear.

It is important to avoid stereotyping people; every culture is complex and diverse. Often, more differences exist between individuals within a particular culture than between the cultures of the patient and doctor. The most important and relevant information about patients' cultures will come from the patients themselves. They are the experts on what cultural uniqueness means to them.

CONCLUSION

Over time, doctors gain an understanding of patients' developmental issues, as well as the proximal and distal contexts in which their patients live their lives. Usually, this information is not gathered in a single encounter as part of a formal social history, but rather is accumulated during many visits that can span numerous months or years. As patient and doctor share life experiences, this understanding becomes richer and more detailed. Knowledge of patients' proximal and distal contexts provides a wealth of understanding with regard to how patients perceive health, respond to disease and experience illness. Finally, understanding the whole person can deepen the physician's knowledge of the human condition, especially the nature of suffering and the responses of persons to sickness (Cassell 1991; Mayeroff 1972).

Preview of the Narratives

The following narratives in this section illustrate the challenges and rewards experienced in understanding the patient as a whole person.

The first narrative, **Chapter 11**, demonstrates how caring for several members of an extended family can assist the physician in understanding complex family dynamics and enhance the provision of care for all family members.

Women who are homeless, use illicit drugs and are sex trade workers are perhaps the most extreme example of how proximal and distal contexts not only impact health but also present major challenges to the patient-doctor relationship. **Chapter 12** serves as a powerful illustration.

The ability to ask for help and share fears regarding the impact of an acute injury on one's work, hobbies and daily activities can be compromised by past experiences and a need to maintain a hard fought sense of independence. The **Chapter 13** narrative provides such a perspective and how the clinician responds with a patient-centered approach.

Chapter 14 helps us gain a greater appreciation of how life experiences dramatically influence how we traverse the final journey to our death. The physician's knowledge of the patient's past experiences and how those experiences dictate how and where she wishes to end her life are invaluable. Furthermore, the physician's sensitivity to the needs of the patient's family helps to provide an end-of-life experience that is both patient- and family-centered.

The narrative in **Chapter 15** also deals with death, in this instance regarding a young boy with muscular dystrophy. His journey is as remarkable as he is. This story reveals how life and death, joy and sorrow are inextricably intertwined. To be part of this family's powerful experience was a privilege for the health care providers who walked with them.

At times the multiple confusion and ensuing chaos of our patients' lives appears foreboding and often hopeless. We seriously question our ability to help. Any hope of resolution, or even the fantasy of a better future, is dashed by their trauma-filled past and their shaky grasp of the present. All these elements come into play in **Chapter 16**, which tells of a young woman whose desolate past and current reality are grim. But in the end, she is victorious.

New beginnings are often difficult. In **Chapter 17**, the sudden loss of a valued therapeutic relationship forces the patient to seek out a new physician. While this creates anxiety for a woman who is already feeling overwhelmed by family caregiving, in the end, it provides her with an unexpected understanding of her context.

Resuscitation in the life of doctors is common. It is extremely technical and driven by strict protocol, but sometimes it can be an unsettling experience. When it's a patient you've known for many years, having experienced their joys and sorrows, it becomes more than just an algorithm. The story in **Chapter 18** exposes the doctor's experience of the last moments of her patient's life and what they mean to her. The story also raises the importance of having family involved in the decision-making process during resuscitation. They are not just onlookers – they are participants.

In **Chapter 19**, we observe how professional ethics forbids a physician to defend the behaviors of his patient either publicly or privately. Therefore, he seeks his catharsis through the telling of her sad and complicated story.

Chapter 20, the final narrative in this section, reveals how a change in an individual's life circumstances altered his experience of being "healthy." It also serves as a segue to the next component of patient-centered care – enhancing the patient-clinician relationship.

Narratives Illustrating Component II:
Understanding the Whole Person

11 Losses and Gains

Lisa Graves and Judith Belle Brown

I inherited 25-year-old Kate as a transfer from a physician who was leaving the city. She came as a package with both of her parents and one of her sisters, who also became my patients.

Stella and Leo, Kate's parents, were fully enmeshed with their daughters' lives. Their eldest, Miriam, had married and moved to the West Coast, where she was a loving, Jewish daughter with a three-hour time change and a costly flight separation from her parents. Kate's younger sister, Jenny, moved out when she started college, and for the past two years had been teaching English in Japan. This left Kate in the role of the "family daughter."

Growing up with Stella and Leo could not have been easy. Their marriage was fraught with discord. Stella found Leo's difficulty in communicating frustrating but understandable. His frequent visits to the casino or to the race track, where he spent more than the family could afford, fueled arguments. While as small business owners the family never really suffered, it was financially tighter than it should have been. It was hard for Stella to be too upset with Leo's lack of communication. Leo was a child of the Holocaust. His parents lived in France during the rise of Nazism. When the inevitable became apparent, they arranged to have Leo hidden as a Catholic student in a boarding school in France. As a young boy of 12, Leo never saw his parents or any other member of his family again. Leo rarely talked about this part of his life. Only in the last five years had he begun to let his family into this portion of his history, and this was only because his life had started to unravel.

Five years ago, Leo and Stella both confronted death head-on. Leo had a successful resection of his colon due to cancer at the same time that Stella was diagnosed with breast cancer. In the light of their threatening illnesses, together they started to peer more deeply into themselves and their family life. They attended couple therapy and were somewhat successful at beginning to diffuse the major problems in their relationship, but the entanglement with their children's lives, and in particular, Kate's, remained.

While both of Kate's parents were battling cancer, Kate and Sam, her husband, became pregnant with their first child. Sam was a solid rock in Kate's life. She had managed to marry the opposite of her parents, and as a couple they were very happy. While Sam did not always appreciate the involvement of his in-laws, he was benignly tolerant of them. The pregnancy was a happy event for the family and provided a buttress against the fear and anxiety of the cancer. Stella attended most of the prenatal appointments with her daughter and was present at her grandson's delivery. Baby Ayden's safe arrival brought joy to a family engulfed by worry. Stella and Leo continued to do well in couple therapy, and they both went into remission. Stella finally admitted to a depression provoked in part by her breast cancer and started medication.

As Ayden grew into a delightful toddler, Kate and Sam planned their second child. Kate's period was late, and an early ultrasound for nuchal translucency revealed a spontaneous miscarriage. Kate recovered well from the D and C, but when six months later, an anticipated pregnancy had not occurred, she became anxious. Kate had a profound sense of her own personal timetable that was not dependent on nature's agenda. Finally, a third pregnancy materialized.

All went well into Kate's pregnancy, and Stella and Leo were delighted because Miriam, their daughter out West, was also due around the same time. Miriam's pregnancy was of some concern, as increased levels of fluid were building up around the baby and an early delivery was planned. Fortunately, the baby was just fine. Stella and Leo travelled to help Miriam with their new grandchild when Kate was 32 weeks pregnant. When Kate appeared for her office visit the day after her parents left for Miriam's, the physician could not detect a fetal heartbeat. An ultrasound confirmed the horrific news. Kate and Sam's baby would be stillborn.

As with all stillbirths, the delivery was a sad event. The delivery itself was easy. Sam and Kate chose not to look at the baby or even know its gender. The baby was buried as per Jewish custom. Kate and Sam remarked at the time that this was in some ways a positive experience for them, as it was the first time they had had to deal with a crisis as a couple. With Kate's parents conveniently away, they felt closer together than before. Medical workup of the still birth suggested antiphospholipid antibody syndrome as a cause, and everyone felt better that at least in this case there was a reason for the poor outcome.

Six months passed after the stillbirth, and Kate became anxious about not conceiving. Kate felt strongly that she could not grieve her stillbirth until she had a new baby in her arms. She implored her perinatalogist for help. Kate was given Clomid, and a triplet pregnancy resulted. On the advice of a new perinatalogist, the pregnancy was reduced to a twin pregnancy. At 18 weeks, Kate started to spot, and despite a short course of bed rest, she delivered her two 18-week-old sons into the toilet at home. The entire family was devastated.

As if things could not get worse, Kate's benign intracranial hypertension, dormant for years, reactivated. Kate mourned the loss of her twins and started again the intensive follow-up to ensure that the increased pressures in her brain did not lead to blindness. Kate agreed to postpone another pregnancy for at least a year. During that year her coagulation disorder stabilized and her benign intracranial hypertension resolved. As Ayden got older, Kate worried about his lack of a sibling, but used the year to get her life back in order. She and Sam even discussed the possibility of no more children. Kate started to make peace with the idea that she had to give up her agenda and accept the lack of control that she had on the events that surrounded her. But Stella and Leo continued to fret over Kate's health.

Finally, Kate became pregnant. The new perinatalogist agreed to follow and deliver the baby. The hematologist gave clearance for Kate to use heparin during pregnancy to reduce the chance of a recurrent loss, and the neurologist gave a clean bill of health regarding her cerebral hypertension. Kate had lost her job due to company downsizing, but the couple took this as a positive sign because she was able to easily attend all of the medical appointments necessitated by her high-risk pregnancy. Kate successfully resisted her mother's attempts to accompany her on these visits. Instead, Sam was at Kate's side. Stella and Leo remained well, and Stella continued her antidepressants, fearing a relapse in the context of her anxiety about Kate's pregnancy and her overall health. To everyone's delight, baby Jade arrived safely and in perfect condition.

As Kate has reflected on events, she feels that she needed to go through all of this to get where she is today. She and Sam delight in their daughter and in their completed family. She has been able to mourn and to let go of her previous losses as well as move forward from an enmeshed relationship with her parents. While she certainly hopes that this is the end of her losses for now, she feels in her own words, "I am ready for whatever life may throw at me!"

12 "I Am Just an Addict – Can I Trust You? – Can You Trust Me?"

Susan Woolhouse and Judith Belle Brown

Her long, straggly brown hair framed her pale, pockmarked face, but her eyes were piercing and unrelentless as 52-year-old Dana bluntly stated, "I've been doing crack for twenty-two years, and it's a habit now. It is a hard and bad habit to break." Dr. Grant sat quietly and listened.

Clearly, the intensity of her drug use had transformed her identity and her life. With pressured speech, Dana stated, "That is just what I do … I am just an addict. This is the only thing I know how to do right now and do it right." For Dana, her need to get high often superseded all her other needs. "This is pretty well all I do, just finding drugs, running around every day doing that. I will do whatever I can to get drugs," she stated flatly. At least Dana was honest about the intensity of her cravings and how her drug use dominated her life, reflected Dr. Grant. But she remained at a loss about how to help Dana.

The next time Dana came to the clinic, Dr. Grant viewed her name with some degree of dread, yet it was mixed with delight – at least Dana had returned. So Dr. Grant tried to sit still and just listen to Dana. Her goal was to engage Dana, not judge her. But it was evident that Dana's isolation due to her drug use contributed to feelings of loneliness.

With an outpouring of uncharacteristic emotion, Dana blurted, "It's scary! Especially if you're by yourself and there's nobody around and you don't know what to do. I am alone, lost, scared, frustrated. I feel like I am in a dark hole and I am never coming up." Dana's eyes were wet with her tears, and her face revealed her deep anguish. "It's not put me in a good place. It put me on the street, and I'm doing stuff I wouldn't normally do if I was not using drugs."

Dr. Grant was overwhelmed by Dana's flood of emotion – this was the first time she had openly revealed the rawness of her feelings. Dana's profound sense of vulnerability, fear and hopelessness were palpable. But Dr. Grant remained at a loss about how to help Dana.

For Dana, using drugs was both a way to escape from the harsh realities of her daily life on the street and to numb her physical and psychological pain. She frankly stated her grim reality: "You feel like you're flying. Like you're in a whole different world. You don't care. You have no feelings. Everything just kind of escapes." Dana paused for a moment, then continued, "but you're kind of lost. But still it is a band-aid to stop the pain." Although Dana had suffered intense physical, social and emotional consequences because of her drug use, she continued to use. How could Dr. Grant help her change this disastrous lifestyle – how could she help Dana?

Over many visits in the months that followed, slowly and with caution, Dana began to reveal her story. "For years I hid from people and didn't answer my phone, didn't answer my door because I was so paranoid. I was just really crazy. I was going insane in my head, 'cause of the drugs. That was how I lived my life. That is still how I live my life, and now I got no home! The stress of it all is getting to me. And you know, stress can play a huge role on your overall health. And it's pretty stressful, this life." Dana's face sunk into her chest.

Over time, as Dana began to trust Dr. Grant, she shared her many losses. They had been devastating and isolating. "I've lost a lot of friends, lost my job, lost my house … I've lost so much," she said. Her voice barely revealed her pain, yet her story expressed her internal anguish. The tragic and violent death of Dana's daughter had precipitated decades of drug use: "I lost a little girl when she was ten. And I've been using ever since." The gravity of that trauma and the multitude of losses she had suffered were so overwhelming and painful for Dana that she had been unable to talk about it with her health care providers. "I just tell them I don't want to talk about it. Which I don't. It's a part of my past," she solemnly expressed.

The desperation to get high overcame Dana's shame at having to participate in the sex trade. She reluctantly shared with Dr. Grant, "I do it sometimes, but I don't want to say much about that. There's not really much I can say about it … I do it, and I don't really enjoy doing it." When Dana had nowhere to sleep, she was often forced to do sexual favors for people in exchange for a roof over her head or use drugs all night to simply stay warm. As Dana explained to Dr. Grant, "Either I had to make money to pay somebody to sleep in their place, or I had to have sex so I could do drugs to stay awake because it's so damn cold outside you have to stay high to stay warm. Man it's a bitch!" While Dana's effect was flat, her body language revealed her frustration and pain with how her life had unfolded.

After several visits over many months, Dana quietly shared with Dr. Grant, "I had to figure you out first. I wasn't able to trust you at first. And I had to trust you before I could open up to you. I knew I could trust you when you said to me, 'Dana, I have all the time you need; I'll just sit here and listen. You tell me what you can.' If I couldn't trust you, then I was saying nothing to you!"

With this tenuous bond of trust established, Dana cautiously considered and then accepted Dr. Grant's suggestion of subsidized housing. It got Dana off the streets – although it was not a perfect solution, it was the first step.

Since being housed, Dana had not needed to work the streets. "And if I go out and do that, I choose to … I rarely do that anymore. I haven't worked the street in over a year. I'm over it."

Dana continued, "I'm more settled now. If I want to use, I know that I can take it home and I know that I can lock my door and the door only opens if I open it."

For Dana, violence was less common in her life, as she didn't have to rely on sex work. Having housing, a significant change in her distal context, had altered her life. "Violence was an everyday thing," she said. Sighing with relief, she added, "but not so much now because now I can just go to my room and shut the door." Her home provided protection from violence and alleviated the need for drugs to numb her pain.

Her pain was not yet over, but perhaps subsiding. Dr. Grant would remain at Dana's side, encouraging each step towards her recovery; ever cognizant that at any moment the process could falter for a multitude of reasons. None the less, Dr. Grant would remain stalwart in her commitment to Dana. Dr. Grant's first goal had been to engage Dana in the relationship – to ascertain her trust – now her long-term goal was to maintain the trust they had worked so hard to establish.

13 The Issue at Hand

Michael Lee-Poy and Judith Belle Brown

While Jacinda Chan, age 45, had been a patient in my practice for over five years, I had only seen her infrequently for minor complaints. The nurse practitioner, affiliated with the practice, had attended to Jacinda's relevant women's health concerns. Jacinda rarely came to see me, so when she had four visits in one month, I suspected something more was troubling her.

Our first visit was focused entirely on the mechanics of her problem. Jacinda noticed a slight pain and a lump on her right forearm six months ago. Thinking nothing of it, she continued her normal routine. However, the pain had become progressively worse and started to hinder her work, her hobbies and her daily activities. The constant ache she carried with her suddenly converted into a shooting pain whenever she rotated her wrist or abducted her thumb.

Jacinda vocalized that she wanted the lump healed, and the pain eradicated. But the tone of her voice and her anxious demeanor implied what she truly longed for – the restoration of her independence – her old self back, with all of its functions and capabilities. Jacinda was a healthy woman with no other medical history and without a pertinent family history. Jacinda was sent for EMG testing to examine her nerve function due to her slow recovery and the severe functional impact. Although slightly decreased, the EMG results were within normal limits. To rule out osteomyelitis, she was also sent for an X-ray, which was negative. Finally, Jacinda was diagnosed with De Quervain's tenosynovitis, an inflammation that involves the synovium and tendons that control the movement of the thumb.

Although we had successfully made a diagnosis and a treatment plan was in place, I was troubled by the fact that I had no idea of who Jacinda was as a person and how this illness experience was altering her life. Despite the fact that we were traveling in unknown territory, I decided to make the journey.

Jacinda was raised in a tumultuous home. Her father, an alcoholic, had physically abused her mother, and they divorced when Jacinda was 10. When describing her childhood, Jacinda would only state that she and her sister had to look after themselves. She never fully divulged the extent of the losses she endured during her childhood, but rather focused on her strength and ability to raise both herself and her younger sister. "Yep, my childhood was tough," Jacinda stated cryptically, with no emotion. "But I got through it okay," she added with pride in her voice.

Jacinda completed high school and found work as a manual laborer in a warehouse. She had been with the company for 25 years and had earned a great deal of respect for her hard work and loyalty. Her job was labor-intensive and required lifting heavy objects, working a forklift, and manual dexterity. Jacinda stated proudly, "I am good at what I do and I love my job." While Jacinda knew she was a valued employee and had seniority, her ongoing illness caused her to fear that her position could be in jeopardy. Financially she was getting by, but she had no savings, and could not afford to lose her job. Jacinda felt diminished in her capabilities and her accomplishments at work. She explained, "I feel ashamed that I can't do the things I did before. When I see my friends who I used to work with, I pretend everything is okay, but I feel so bad that I can't work with them like I used to."

Jacinda had married when she was 20 years old, and she and her husband had one daughter. Her marriage, like that of her parents, did not fare well, and as a result Jacinda had been single for almost two decades. She was close to her daughter, who was away at college. However, not wanting to upset her daughter with the news of her deteriorating health, Jacinda had not shared her concerns. "She is getting straight A's in all her courses," said Jacinda with a mother's fierce pride. "I don't want to worry her, because she needs to focus on her studies."

Jacinda loved to work in her perennial garden, and she was an avid quilter; in fact, some of her beautiful quilts had received top honors at the local fall fairs. Both hobbies were now severely compromised by her wrist pain. "I used to enjoy gardening so much, but I can't do it anymore," she said with deep resignation in her voice.

Jacinda explained that most of the time she just sat around and watched television, because she could not do anything else. Previously a very active person, she found watching television boring, extremely sedentary and limiting. Her frustration was blatantly obvious as she stated, "I sit and watch TV because it's not like there is anything else I can do, but then I get this antsy feeling, and I turn it off, stand up, pace around for a while, try to do something, and realize I can't, and then plop right back down and turn on the TV again." Although Jacinda didn't say it, you could hear the defeat in her voice. She had tried to deny the impact the pain was having on her life, but it was obvious that she was deeply affected by her limitations.

After a few visits, Jacinda admitted, though hesitantly, that she was feeling quite down. But as a person who prided herself on being independent and having managed on her own for many years, she dismissed her sadness. "Well that is to be expected. I'll manage. I always have." But through her words, I could hear her frustration, her disappointment, her loss. A part of her was broken, and Jacinda had not been able to resolve it on her own. This threatened a part of her identity she cherished – her independence. While Jacinda's independence was a great asset, it was also a hindrance, as it prevented her from seeking help, or even considering relying on another person. Jacinda's frustration and sense of dependence was reaching her upper limit of tolerance. "There are times I feel so hopeless … why has it taken so long? What am I doing wrong?" she asked wearily.

Only in a later visit did she reveal her true fears. She broke down. "I am so sorry you have to see me this way," she sobbed at the beginning of the encounter, "I don't like people to see me crying." After a short pause, Jacinda revealed, "I've been crying almost every day when I get home. I can control myself at work, and then when I get home I can't stop crying." For the first time, Jacinda admitted the depth of her feelings. We talked some more and agreed it was okay for her to recognize her sadness and express it. After a few more tears and a quiet, reflective pause, Jacinda revealed her ultimate fear: "What if I never get better?" We sat there in silence, me not knowing what to say, and Jacinda realizing the true extent of her loss.

In the beginning, Jacinda had been reluctant to ask for help, as she was not accustomed to sharing her feelings with others. But as our relationship evolved and we got Jacinda through this health crisis, she became more at ease. While Jacinda remained a woman of few words, her ability to ask for help was no longer a threat to her independence.

By learning more about Jacinda as a person, I came to understand how her past life experiences influenced her current response to being unwell. I also recognized how difficult it was for her to ask for help and to share her feelings. She felt scared and ashamed as her independence rapidly eroded. An important part of our plan was to restore her confidence and help her regain her independence. Had I not known her past challenges in life, I could have easily misinterpreted her response to her illness and as such not fully understood the magnitude of her problem.

14 "I Want to Die at Home"

Michelle Levy and Judith Belle Brown

Dr. Solomon had always looked forward to his visits with his patient Nadia Castire. A bright and energetic woman, she appeared younger than her 82 years. Nadia was the proud mother of four grown children and a boastful grandmother of six. During her 60-year marriage to Rowland, they had shared the joys and sorrows of raising a family. All this had been revealed to Dr. Solomon over the 20 years he had been their family physician. Dr. Solomon shook his head in disbelief. It had only been two months since Nadia had been diagnosed with advanced cancer. And now she was gone.

Nadia had initially presented with general malaise, weakness and decreased appetite approximately eight weeks earlier. A non-tender abdominal mass was suspicious upon examination, plus Nadia was jaundiced. Abdominal ultrasound and subsequent CT were suggestive of a cholangiocarcinoma (Klatskin tumor). The opinion of the consulting gastroenterologist was that this was an advanced tumor, with significant local spread – surgery was not an option. Nadia was then seen by oncology to determine if palliative chemotherapy or radiation would be of any benefit for symptom control and to improve her quality of life. Unfortunately, these were also determined not to be an option.

Nadia received each piece of bad news with stoicism. Yet, she found it hard to reconcile how everything had moved so rapidly since her initial diagnosis. However, Nadia was not interested in any treatment that could potentially make her feel worse during the little time she had left. She calmly stated, "I really appreciate how everyone is being straight with me, as I wouldn't want to do anything that could make me more sick, even if it meant being around a little longer. I want whatever time I have left to be quality time with my family."

Accompanied by her husband Rowland, she had come to Dr. Solomon's office over the next few weeks. Each time she appeared more weak, yet determined to walk unattended, albeit more slowly. Nadia's major concern symptomatically was her persistent pruritus. It had improved slightly, as had her jaundice, after a biliary stent was placed. However, it still affected her sleep, and she was getting excoriations from scratching. She found the various antipruritic medications somewhat helpful at night since they made her sleepy, but she was generally avoiding them during the day. Nadia had little appetite, but she had said, smiling, "This is more concerning to my family than to me!"

Nadia was a happy and content person, who even prior to her illness, always tended to minimize her symptoms. Dr. Solomon had always viewed Nadia as a very intelligent and well-organized woman. Prior to this illness, she would come to follow–up appointments for her blood pressure armed with charts and graphs she created on her computer. An independent woman, Nadia had wanted to do as much as possible for herself. She had a very strong faith and went to church every week. This was of comfort to her and she stated, "I am not afraid to die." She also wanted to die at home.

Dr. Solomon had not known Nadia when she worked as a nurse at the local long-term care facility, but he certainly was well-versed on her opinions about such institutions. So it was no surprise to Dr. Solomon when Nadia adamantly stated, "I want to die at home." Over the years, Nadia had shared with Dr. Solomon how she had observed "many poor souls who wouldn't want to be alive if they only knew." Nadia had seen too many people who had lived like "vegetables" for years in the long-term care facility, and wanted to make sure she wasn't one of them. Thus, Nadia's professional life as a nurse in a long-term care facility served as a major influence on her decision regarding where she wished to die. Indeed, these distant, yet powerful memories only increased her intent to remain at home and not be forced to move into a long-term care facility near the end.

Soon, office visits to Dr. Solomon became home visits in order for Dr. Solomon to assess how both Nadia and Rowland were coping. Nadia's most prominent issue was the desire to be in control of the decision-making surrounding the goals for her care and treatment priorities, including where she was to die. Dr. Solomon reassured her that whether at home or at the hospice, only comfort care measures would be taken to make sure she was as pain- and symptom-free as possible. He also explained that the very nature of her illness suggested her time at the hospice would be brief. Nadia indicated she would be willing to go to hospice if, together, they felt it was "almost over" and if it was getting too difficult for Rowland to care for her at home. Rowland and her children were committed to fulfilling Nadia's wish to remain home until the end. Yet Dr. Solomon soberly noted how Rowland appeared exhausted and emotionally drained. Community resources were enlisted and altogether they began Nadia's palliative care journey.

Nadia's condition rapidly deteriorated. She was very concerned about taking any medication, fearful they might alter her thinking – she did not want to feel out of control. Dr. Solomon encouraged Nadia to share how she was feeling physically, mentally, emotionally and spiritually so together they could determine how to best manage her symptoms and provide her optimal comfort.

While Nadia already seemed to have found some peace of mind in openly dealing with her feelings about life and death, she continued to fear the loss of control that could result with symptomatic treatment. Nadia shared her anxiety about becoming a burden on her family and at the same time worried how her husband of 60 years would manage without her. Nadia and Rowland had a loving and supportive relationship. It would be hard to say goodbye. In addition, her faith and religious beliefs continued to be of solace to her.

Dr. Solomon was also concerned that if Nadia stayed at home instead of coming to the hospice near the end, it would be difficult to maintain symptom control and pain relief. He too worried about the toll on 85-year-old Rowland's health. Unlike Nadia, he had not been immune to serious health issues in the past, having suffered two heart attacks in his late-70s, as well as the onset of type 2 diabetes. Rowland's health was fragile, and for years the focus had been on him. But now this was Nadia's time.

In the end, a few days before her death, Nadia was transferred to a hospice. Although she was becoming more confused, Nadia was able to clearly and independently make the decision regarding this transition in her care. She was concerned because Rowland had not slept in days and was on the brink of collapse. Even with the daily nursing support and family help, Nadia knew they were no longer able to manage at home. The time had come.

Dr. Solomon met with Nadia and her family for the next two days at the hospice. As Nadia slipped in and out of consciousness, they all reminisced about her life and the love she had extended to her family, friends and patients. Dr. Solomon was grateful for having known this fine woman for 20 years. It had been a privilege to care for her and to be present during this final passage of her life. Nadia died peacefully the following evening in her sleep, surrounded by her family and in the presence of her family physician.

15 A Young Boy's Journey

Sharon Nur Hatcher

The story I am about to tell you is one of the most profound and significant experiences in my work as a family doctor. I first met Jeremy when I followed his mother's pregnancy with her third child. Jeremy was the oldest at the age of seven, followed by his sister, who was five years old at the time. Jeremy's mother, Clara, told me of her son, who suffered from a severe mutated form of Duchenne muscular dystrophy. Genetic testing of family members was negative, and subsequent children were unlikely to be affected. The prognosis for Jeremy was very poor – he was unlikely to reach adulthood.

The family lived on a farm in the country, and their home served as temporary housing for unwed teenage mothers. Jeremy's father, Rene, also had a job as a gardener in order to supplement the family's income. I was immediately struck by the poignancy of this family situation, their serenity and their courage. I started visiting the family once a month to provide holistic care for all of them, accompanying the family members as they faced this incredible journey.

Jeremy was diagnosed at two-and-a-half years of age after a painful muscle biopsy. He still was not walking and had been hypotonic as well as developmentally delayed since infancy. By three-and-a-half years of age, Jeremy could walk but showed symptoms of autism, and he was also diagnosed with epilepsy. Jeremy spent the next year and a half attending the day hospital at the regional psychiatric institute for intensive therapy. Over time, his social skills improved and normalized, his epilepsy no longer needed treatment and he was able to attend a specialized school near the family farm.

When I met Jeremy, at the age of seven he could no longer walk; instead, he used an electric wheelchair that he enjoyed zooming around in. He was very alert and interested in everything going on around him: the garden, the animals and his little sister, who would hop on the back of his wheelchair for a ride. Jeremy's room had been adapted to his needs, with many toys positioned on custom-made shelves at wheelchair height, as well as a special lift to get him in and out of his bath. Jeremy was very bright and inquisitive, asking constant questions that required satisfactory answers. He knew about the nature of his disease. His parents were open about the fact that he would die someday.

I had decided to come and meet Jeremy in his home to get to know him and to evaluate the family situation. Jeremy was followed regularly by a clinic that specialized in muscular dystrophy. He would often be hospitalized on the pediatric floor with infections such as pneumonia and gastroenteritis. Although the family was very creative in finding ways to provide Jeremy with as much of a normal life as possible, his parents often felt overwhelmed by his progressive deterioration. With fear and anxiety, they anticipated what was to come.

Over the next few years, Jeremy deteriorated rapidly. By the age of 11, he had lost 50% of his lung capacity, had severe scoliosis and could barely sit up. His parents were told that little else could be done for him and to prepare for the worst. Jeremy became extremely anxious and would wake up screaming from nightmares. In the midst of her suffering, his mother would recount: "We had lost the meaning of his life, of our lives, we had completely lost control."

Clara and I came to realize how everyone's life in the family had been put on hold as they all waited for Jeremy's imminent death. But he didn't die – he got *better*, at least in spirit. A decision was made to stop going to the hospital for specialized care and instead to treat him at home if he got an infection. Two years of relative peaceful stability followed. Jeremy was happy, he ate and slept well. He rarely got sick. He insisted on going to school. He became an adolescent with pubertal changes in his emaciated body. By the age of 13, he was about four feet long and weighed 40 lbs. But Jeremy's spirit was soaring. He managed to attend six months of high school, mostly on a stretcher. He fell in love with a girl in his class. Jeremy made plans for his future.

On several occasions his mother confided to me that even when she was a few weeks pregnant with Jeremy, she had an intuition that he would be different. "I knew he would have a special gift, but would also suffer a lot," she said with raw emotion. Indeed, throughout his short life, Jeremy greatly influenced the people he encountered. Some were perfect strangers who would be so affected by the presence of this child that their lives were totally transformed.

One such occasion occurred when Jeremy was 10 years old. He had learned about Picasso in art class at school. He then painted a picture on the back of a pizza box. Jeremy brought it home to show his mom, who put it aside. Indeed, she almost threw it out. Shortly afterward, some artist friends were visiting and noticed the picture. They were taken with the depth and symbolism in the abstract painting. They could see the outline of a wheelchair as well as a galloping horse. There were dark and bright colors. There were the trees and the forest, as well as the light of the heavens. The painting was shown to an art gallery owner in a nearby city. Thus the work, entitled

"The Secret," became part of an exhibition at the gallery. It was reproduced and sold to raise money for muscular dystrophy. Clara considered this painting to be Jeremy's final testament.

The last year of Jeremy's life was eventful and difficult. He was 14 and completely bedridden. He developed bedsores. He was in pain and had difficulty sleeping. He needed constant care. Home care was supplemented by a few close friends. He took pain and sleep medication but also had side effects such as urinary retention and severe constipation. He developed a gastrointestinal ulcer from the anti-inflammatory medication. He ate less and less. He choked on secretions but could not tolerate a suction machine. End-of-life decisions were discussed. His parents wanted him to die at home. We all agreed that there would be no oxygen or ventilator support to prolong his suffering.

The last year brought another surprise: an unexpected pregnancy for Clara at the age of 40. I still remember her in my office, utterly devastated. She was exhausted with chronic sorrow and couldn't imagine how she could get through the pregnancy, let alone take care of a baby. Her inner resources were depleted despite her strong faith. Once Clara got over her initial shock, she and her husband decided to pursue the pregnancy. At first, she had excessive energy but spent the last month in bed because of back strain from lifting Jeremy. As their family physician, I had the unique experience of carrying out concurrent prenatal care for one child while doing palliative care for another – all in the same family. The baby was born in May and Jeremy died in August, on his 15th birthday.

That day had been a happy one. Jeremy had not eaten or drank for five days and was receiving regular morphine injections. But he insisted on celebrating his birthday and even tried, unsuccessfully, to blow out the candles on his birthday cake. That night, he woke up his mother and whispered, "Mommy, I'm fine. Mommy, thank you. Mommy, I love you." Then he slipped gently away.

When I arrived at their home I remember the tremendous sense of peace and serenity that greeted me in the silence of the night. Jeremy's parents awoke the other children to say goodbye to their older brother. They took turns carrying his withered and twisted body around the house, trying to let him go. His funeral was simple and very moving. White balloons were released into the sky and I remember seeing a rainbow. Jeremy had an angelic presence for so many people in their times of difficulty.

Five years have passed, and the family has managed to continue without the physical presence of Jeremy. But it has been a painful and sometimes uneven process of grieving and healing. I for one, as their family physician, feel so privileged to have been allowed to be part of such a journey, and it continues.

16 Victor Brings Victory

Larry Schmidt and Judith Belle Brown

The women's clinic was buzzing with activity as the patients shuffled in for their antenatal care. The low-risk obstetrical clinic was designed to service primarily women who did not have access to a family physician. Most of the patients were relatively uncomplicated, but some were not.

My first impression when I walked into the examining room was that there was no one in the room. As I was about to leave the room, with my hand on the door, I realized that my patient was in the room. *"How odd,"* I thought as I checked the chart. She was curled up in the fetal position tucked in behind the examination room door. She was all dressed in black and blue streaked hair hid her face.

Before me I saw a very traumatized 19-year-old woman who looked absolutely frightened for her life. She was obviously pregnant as she cringed in the corner hugging her frail body, refusing to make eye contact or speak. "Hello Reese," I said as I began the introductions. She seemed to curl up even tighter. This clearly was the challenge of the day, and I proceeded to commence a monologue of what my responsibility to her could be and what she could be doing in the interim between this and our next visit.

Slowly Reese appeared to relax and her body began to unfurl. I continued on telling her that she looked approximately 26 weeks pregnant and hopefully we could engage in a therapeutic relationship that might help her in the long run. I acknowledged how her body language seemed to suggest that she was a traumatized young woman and perhaps there were things we could help her with here at the clinic. I also mentioned that we had a full-time social worker at the clinic who is available Friday mornings. Reese remained silent throughout the encounter with her head hung low. She left the room looking angry and fearful and, in spite of my best efforts, I did not expect I would ever see her again.

Much to my amazement, Reese appeared in the clinic two weeks later. When I walked into the room she was sitting in a chair and not behind the door. Reese looked upwards on several occasions to see what I looked like and, on a few occasions, engaged in conversation, albeit very tentatively. "Reese," I said as the visit came to a close, "I would like you to see me on a weekly basis, as there is much to catch up on to make your pregnancy safe and healthy."

"Okay," responded Reese in her familiar monosyllabic manner.

Over the next many weeks Reese gradually opened up and shared some of her past medical history. Not only had she been traumatized by many people in her life but also by health care providers who did not take the time to find out where her vulnerabilities lay. As Reese's story unfolded, a dysfunctional family history was revealed. She grew up in an alcoholic family that moved around a great deal, and her parents separated when she was 12. Reese lived with her father, while her two elder brothers had remained with her mother. Reese described a very acrimonious relationship with her mother. "She always accused me of going with the wrong crowd," explained Reese, "So I did just to piss her off!" Reese dropped out of school in grade 11 and either couch surfed or lived on the street. Sadly, she continued, "There was no love in my family."

Reese was raped at age 15, and her father was far from supportive. With her jaw tightly clenched, Reese bluntly stated, "He told me I probably deserved it." This rape came to light during discussions around why Reese found it difficult to have blood work drawn. Her previous family physician, who had looked after her for the early part of her pregnancy, had grabbed her arm and told her not to be such a baby. Reese flashed back to the rape she experienced at the hands of her uncle. "Don't be such a baby" were the exact same words her uncle used while he raped her. Reese had suffered several other sexual assaults since the initial rape at age 15.

After many visits and the development of a therapeutic relationship, Reese did have a successful delivery of a male infant. It is noteworthy that during the delivery process, Reese frequently disempowered herself by imploring us to pull the baby out. "Get it out of me," she cried as the contractions shook her small frame. But I refused. "You have to push the baby out Reese," I said, "I am here as an assistant in your birthing process. This is your baby to deliver."

After the birth of her son, Reese began to withdraw into her former self. She lay curled up in a fetal position in her hospital bed and one-word answers returned. Attempts at breastfeeding were abysmal, and she expressed ambivalence about naming her baby. "Every name I come up with reminds me of some guy who's jerked me around in the past," she lamented.

Reese deferred to the nurses in her newborn's care. She muttered, "I don't know how to bathe him." They became increasingly concerned about the lack of bonding between mother and child and notified the antenatal social worker. She in turn, fulfilling her professional obligations, contacted child protective services. Institutional chaos ensued. I was out of my depth in this situation, but what happened to Reese and her baby did matter to me. She had made such gains, and I couldn't let her falter. Reese deserved some success in her life.

But, unknown to me was the role child protective services had played in Reese' childhood. It all surfaced now as her role as a mother was in jeopardy. Throughout her chaotic childhood, Reese and her brothers had bounced in and out of foster care, sometimes together but often apart. Another shard of Reese's past had been exposed.

Calm returned as plans were made for Reese and her baby regarding housing and postpartum care. Child protective services, awash with more challenging cases, rapidly discharged Reese into the social service abyss. But my concerns remained. Reese, now at age 20, was unemployed with no job in sight and had minimal social supports. She was managing to care for her little baby boy, named Victor – to reflect his victorious future, as Reese proclaimed and this was her sole focus. I saw her as vulnerable and at risk of virtually replicating the disaster of her family of origin.

I had to find a way to help Reese. Somehow we had to create a future path that was different from the horrible journey she had travelled in her past.

After what felt like an inordinate amount of coaxing and cajoling, we finally found common ground. Reese agreed to meet with Deanna, the social worker. Much to her surprise, and my relief, Reese liked Deanna. "She gets me," said Reese triumphantly. Soon they began meeting weekly to address the many challenging elements of Reese's life – finding better housing, securing subsidized daycare, finding help with transportation costs, completing her high school education. But most of all they talked, and Reese poured out years of sorrow and emotional neglect. In Deanna she found someone who would listen to her, someone who didn't find her past abhorrent, and someone who wasn't going to judge her. During this time, I for the most part stood in the wings watching Reese grow and mature. I would see her occasionally for some minor ailment, and of course routine well baby checks.

I marvel at how Reese has hurdled all the obstacles that she has faced. At times they have seemed insurmountable to me, and I can only imagine what they have felt to her. But she has done it, against all the odds. She is victorious.

17 New Beginnings

Barbara Jones, Judith Belle Brown and Tanya Thornton

Although Margaret had been here on dozens of occasions before, this was a new experience for her. Margaret sat nervously rotating the rings on her finger as she glanced around the busy waiting room. "Margaret?" the nurse called from the doorway. In an instant she was standing and heading to meet her new doctor.

As Margaret settled into the chair in the examining room, she smoothed her plaid skirt and tried to relax. *"This is silly,"* she reflected to herself, *"I am a fifty-four-year-old adult, but I'm acting like an anxious twelve year old!"* But then the feeling flooded back. *"How could he retire?"* she thought. *"He'd been my doctor for thirty years, delivered my two children, supported me when dad died five years ago from that awful stroke, and then 'poof,' just like that, he shuts down his practice,"* Margaret ruminated. Now she had to start all over again with a new doctor.

A knock on the door interrupted her thoughts.

"Hello Margaret! Good to see you again," said Dr. Hass cheerily as she entered the room.

"Hello, Doctor, thanks for agreeing to see me," Margaret replied.

Dr. Hass had first met Margaret two years ago, when her 80-year-old mother, Roma, was found to have a large ovarian cancer. She experienced serious postoperative complications and never fully recovered. Roma subsequently required chemotherapy in a specialized center and moved into Margaret's home during her treatment. Two years later, she was still living with her daughter. Roma's health was showing some decline as of late. She was now incontinent, somewhat confused at times, and unable to read or do any fine work as a result of the postoperative complications. She was also unsteady on her feet and unable to negotiate the stairs in the house, making her effectively housebound.

Prior to this visit, Dr. Hass had seen Margaret on many occasions with her mother and had visited them at home, but she had never seen Margaret on her own.

"So, Margaret," asked Dr. Hass, "how can I help you today?"

As Margaret took a deep breath, she could feel the tears sting her eyes. *"Get a grip on yourself,"* she thought admonishingly. "Well," she began, "as you may know, Dr. Kahn has retired and I need a new doctor."

"Yes, I did hear about his retirement," Dr. Hass replied.

"I just got a letter telling me he was closing the practice. There had been no indication at my last visit with him, a month ago, that he might be leaving. Then suddenly he's gone." Margaret paused momentarily, and as she continued she could feel her face begin to flush. "I had known him for years and had good relationship with him, or so I thought."

"It sounds as if it was quite a shock for you," observed Dr. Hass.

"Yes, yes it was," said Margaret, her emotions barely beneath the surface, "I trusted him with my care, and then he abandoned me," Margaret began to quietly weep.

Dr. Hass passed Margaret a Kleenex and said, "You seem very upset by his retirement."

"It's the thought of starting all over again with a new doctor that I find so difficult," said Margaret wiping her tears.

"I'd be happy to take over your care if you are comfortable with that arrangement," offered Dr. Hass.

"Thank you, doctor," replied Margaret with a sigh of relief.

"Tell me a little about what's happening with you currently," inquired Dr. Hass.

Margaret took another deep breath. "Well, as you know, mother's health is continuing to decline."

"Yes," nodded Dr. Hass, "In the past our focus has always been on your mother, but how are you doing?"

As Margaret's story unfolded, Dr. Hass learned that part of her current problems were related to her mother's illness – she found it very stressful looking after Roma. Her life had been limited by not being able to leave her mother unattended for any length of time, and her relationship with her husband was feeling the strain. Margaret felt somewhat guilty that she had been making inquires about long-term care for her mother, but as she explained, "I feel like I have no choice." Her mother was incontinent, a stressing situation for them both, as Roma had always been very fastidious about her personal hygiene. Margaret wondered how much longer she would be able to care for her mother as she became more frail. "I wonder what I will be like when I am her age," she concluded.

While much of her life has been devoted to the care of others, Margaret did feel she should have interests of her own and was beginning to enjoy the freedom of not having children at home before her mother moved in with her. Margaret had been very devoted to her mother and wished to care for her but found she was not able to continue to do so, especially as her siblings did not help much. Her brother took Roma for a day a month, and one sister visited every two weeks. She was unhappy with their lack of support, and felt resentful that the burden of responsibility fell upon her shoulders. Her husband felt she had done more than enough for her mother and that it was time for her to be placed in a long-term care facility. "I know my husband is right," sighed Margaret, "but when I visit those various nursing homes I just feel so guilty about putting mother in such a place." It was clear that Margaret felt torn between her loyalty to her husband and her loyalty to her mother.

Margaret's life had contracted drastically since assuming her mother's care. Margaret had given up her church activities to be with her mother. "I really miss singing in the choir. It was such a pleasure," Margaret said with regret. Her friends now visited infrequently, as it was awkward with her mother. Her greatest loss was not being able to spend time with her young grandchildren. "They are such a delight," she stated, smiling proudly, "and they are at that precious age. Oh I do miss them, but I can't leave mother to go visit them." Her sadness was readily apparent.

The second major issue for Margaret was the loss of her relationship with her doctor. His sudden retirement had been a serious blow for her. Dr. Hass felt fortunate that she already had some contact with Margaret and certainly now had a better understanding of her context. The challenge would be to gain her confidence and trust.

"Margaret," said Dr. Hass as the visit concluded, "there is certainly a lot of stress associated with caring for your mother. I can see that it is causing distress and perhaps we need to talk further about how together we might make some changes that are good for both of you. What do you think?"

"Oh that would be wonderful! I do feel overwhelmed by all the responsibility," replied Margaret. The sound of relief filled the air.

A new patient-doctor relationship was beginning.

18 The Onlookers

Rochelle Dworkin, Judith Belle Brown and Tanya Thornton

"Dr. Leung, the ICU is paging you, Mr. Larcouix is in respiratory distress!" The nurse's voice was out there somewhere on the other end of the phone, but my sleep-deprived hearing was having trouble registering her words in the wonderful blackness of slumber. "Dr. Leung! Dr. Leung, Mr. Lacrouix –"

"Yes, yes, I heard you – I'm coming." I yawned, turning on the call-room light and hanging up the phone. I peered at my watch – it was 1:00 a.m. I had left the ICU only 30 minutes ago and all was fine. I had hoped for at least a couple of hours of sleep to refresh my brain, but alas, it would have to wait. I threw the sheets off, grabbed my stethoscope and forced myself up out of bed. By the time I hit the brightly lit hallways, I was awake enough to run. Out of breath when I entered the ICU, I almost ran into Eva, Mr. Marshall Lacrouix's wife, who was opening the door in a rush to the unit.

"How is he – I came as fast as I could. Is he okay?" Eva poured out.

"He's having trouble breathing," I replied, leading the way to his cubicle. As I pulled back the privacy curtain around his bed, I suddenly realized Mr. Lacrouix was in trouble. His hands and lips had turned a dusky purple, and he was thrashing about, confused, gasping for air. I looked up at the monitor. His oxygen level was too low to sustain him much longer. "We have to intubate, get the cart ready," I ordered. I turned to Eva, still standing in the doorway, fear evident in her eyes. "Eva, I need to put a tube down his throat to help him breathe, is that okay? He's too confused right now to tell me his wishes. Is that what he would want?"

"Yes! Do everything you can, Dr. Leung. I'm not ready to lose him yet."

Sometime between intubation and thrombolysis, the rest of Mr. Lacrouix's family members arrived. When I looked up to again gain permission to use a clot-busting medicine to treat his heart attack, I found myself facing Eva, surrounded by their four children and their spouses. As Eva lovingly stroked Marshall's cold hand, she replied, "Yes, please do all you can."

"There's a risk that, because of his recent surgery, he may have a life-threatening bleed from the medicine that we use to try to break up the clot around his heart. Is that risk okay with you Eva?"

"But if you don't try, he will likely die – right?"

"Yes, it is very possible."

With her son's hands on her shoulders, she looked me in the eye. "Treat the heart attack. Our family needs him."

"Okay." I smiled, giving her arm a quick gentle squeeze as I walked to the head of the bed.

The nurses had already prepared the medication. It was the start of the end. It was also a beginning.

Mr. Lacrouix was a 76-year-old man who had undergone surgery one week earlier for a small bowel obstruction. Although his post-operative course had been medically complicated, he had finally stabilized and was going to be transferred to the floor the following morning, until the advent of his acute respiratory distress. Within 30 minutes of the onset of his shortness of breath, his family witnessed aggressive management of cardiogenic shock, cardiac arrest and a full resuscitation.

When it became evident that Mr. Lacrouix was dead, I reached out to touch Eva's arm. "He's gone Eva. I'm so sorry. There is nothing more we can do now." I paused. Silence enveloped the room. "Would you like us to stop the chest compressions?"

She continued to stroke his forehead and then leaned in for a final kiss. Without looking up, she nodded yes, as the first tear dropped on his gray cheek.

I saw her son's eyes follow my gaze to the clock as I called out the time. "Time of death 1:32 a.m." I turned to Eva. "Please stay as long as you want. Take your time saying goodbye to Marshall. Just let the nurse know when you are done." I brought a stool over for Eva. She sat down, never taking her eyes off Marshall.

I left the room in silence. The nurses understood somehow that they were to give the family as much privacy as needed, although we never spoke the words. There was the disappointment that comes after an unsuccessful resuscitation but it was overshadowed by an inner peace and contentment that I had never experienced before. Having practiced emergency medicine in this small town for nearly 20 years, I had left many unsuccessful resuscitations, but this one was different. This was not the typical "Code Blue" at our hospital. It was the first time in the history of the hospital, and the first time in my experience, that the patient's family was in attendance throughout the resuscitation and for the final minutes of a life.

On reflection, I became cognizant of how appropriate and comforting it felt to have Mr. Lacrouix's family present during his final minutes. Regardless of the numerous onlookers, the ICU felt ordered and calm. More importantly, the family's presence facilitated the decision-making process along the way. Despite the outcome, the family witnessed and understood that everything possible had been attempted. In the end, this would be healing for both family and physician.

Mr. Lacrouix was not just a patient in extremis for me. I had treated him several times while on duty in the emergency room. I had delivered one of his grandchildren and had mourned with his daughter when her husband died suddenly at a young age only months after their baby was born. I knew of the active role Mr. Lacrouix played in our small community as a well-respected businessman and leader of many charities. Knowing how important he was to his family, and they to him, made it feel all the more natural that they should be with him during the final minutes of his life.

We speak of the patient-physician relationship, yet this does not exist in isolation. It behooves every treating physician to remember that the patient being resuscitated is usually part of a family and a member of a community. We need to recognize the existence of two patients in this situation: the one in the resuscitation room and the one(s) in the quiet room, the family – both seeking help and both suffering. Traditionally, we have neglected to perceive this, as we are busy "running a code." Families influence health, and health and illness influence families. Including the family validates the experience for them.

In all human interactions, an inherent complexity exists – none as prominent as in the resuscitative context. We must recognize it and respond. It has been our duty throughout our professional practice, and we should not abandon this responsibility at the time of death. Attention and presence to both patient and family afford us "success" where little fruition is conceivable.

19 The Criminal

Peter MacKean, Judith Belle Brown and Tanya Thornton

Tulips were beginning to bloom, and there was a freshness in the air marking the arrival of spring. My step was brisk as I entered the hospital for morning rounds.

"Got a new one for you, doc! A real gem," the nurse said, handing me a hospital chart. "Angela Witmer, 38 years old, admitted to the psych ward last night with a diagnosis of homicidal ideation." The nurse paused to scan her clipboard, "Oh, it says here you're her GP – you must know all about her then."

"I know Angela," I replied. At least, I thought I knew her. After all, I had been her family physician for the past 25 years, but her diagnosis seemed surreal to me.

When I arrived on the ward, I was quickly ushered into a private room by a police officer. He enthusiastically pronounced, "We're charging her with several offenses. Last evening she was seen driving recklessly down the road. After she screeched into the parking lot of her husband's business, she crashed into his car and stormed into his office, yelling, 'Why are you doing this to me?' His coworkers said that she was completely out of control and was in such a rage that they thought she might kill him. When we arrived, her breathalyzer was high and she was combative, so we cuffed her." He smirked, "We know that she's here involuntarily under the mental health act, so don't let her go without calling us."

With these 'facts' in tow, I entered Angela's room. She looked up from her hospital bed, hair askew, eyes still glazed from the lingering effects of alcohol.

"I don't know how it came to this," she began, sobbing. "Yes, things were bad between Mark and I, and I'm extremely angry with him – who wouldn't be! He took everything from me: our home, my job, but most of all, it's our girls that I've lost. But I never wanted to hurt him!" As quickly as her revelation began, it ceased. "I want to be alone – please leave."

At the office later that day, my first patient said, "Did you hear about Angela Witmer? I guess she went berserk and tried to kill her husband last night … what a way to treat a man who is now raising their two children alone. She's a deranged woman who deserves to be locked up, once she gets out of the loony bin." With that, he rose and left the office. Had he come in for medical advice, or just to voice his opinion? Did he know I was her family physician? I was startled by his reaction, even more so than the actual events of the night in question. As her family physician, I had known Angela since she was a teenager and did not see her as a criminal. Of course, my professional ethics forbade me from defending her publicly or privately.

Although the community would never know her past, I bore the privileged knowledge that Angela had been raped by an uncle when she was seven and had been emotionally and physically abused by her own father. She and her mother escaped to our peaceful community to start a new life. Unfortunately, Angela found solace in alcohol and street drugs. As is common in those who have been abused, she became hypersexual. At age 16 she became pregnant, insisted on an abortion and quit high school.

At her mother's insistence, she enrolled in a secretarial training program and graduated upon completion of the program. This was the first time in her life that she felt that she had succeeded in anything. I remember her bouncing into the office with pride in her voice, telling me, "I did it, doc! I really did it! I graduated with honors. Now I can get a real job and start my life."

"*What has happened to that Angela,*" I wondered.

Harry happened, and then Mark. Harry became Angela's first husband, the father of her firstborn – Joshua – and the first to break her heart, when he was found having an affair with a co-worker. She became a single mother and resumed drinking. She secured a bank loan to start a small business in her home, which allowed her to spend more time with her young son. It was around this time that she met Mark, a local builder. Their relationship flourished and a year later, they married and had two daughters: Lindsay Joan and Erika Ann – the pride of their lives.

Everything seemed to be going well. Although still considered an outcast by older people in the community, her salon business was becoming more popular among younger girls, who were looking for more trendy styles. As for Mark, his contracting business expanded rapidly. The children were growing. Joshua was now 16, Lindsay 12 and Erika nine.

A week before that fateful night at Mark's office, Lindsay approached Angela after school. "Mommy, what does rape mean?" Lindsay inquired innocently. At first, Angela wasn't sure how to answer, so she consulted a brochure entitled "How to talk to your children about sex." She asked Lindsay to read the appropriate piece on rape. After reviewing it, Lindsay looked up and said, "Rape … I think that's what's happening to me." Angela tried, but couldn't contain her horror. With thoughts of her own rape hitting her like a thunderbolt, she searched for answers.

"Mom, he told me not to tell you," Lindsay said with tears of shame, "but Josh has been raping me for the last two years."

When Josh came home that night, he was grilled by Angela. He admitted to everything, and over the next 24 hours, complete chaos enveloped their home. Angela banished Joshua from their family.

Lindsay pursued counseling. Angela turned to vodka. In the same week, she lost her dream occupation, grieved her daughter's violation and saddled herself with lifelong guilt. Mark blamed her for not protecting "their" daughter from "her" son.

In the end, Mark and Angela separated. One evening, a physical fight ensued while Angela was drinking. In the altercation, Angela punched Mark in the face and the police were called. She was forced out of the home, served with a restraining order and allowed only telephone access to her daughters. Without access to her hairdressing equipment, she was unemployed and forced to stay at her mother's house. She desperately missed her daughters and felt bitter about Mark's unfair treatment of her. Angela began drinking heavily again, sank into a deep depression and constantly thought about suicide. With Angela's anger becoming more intense and with the alcohol clouding her thinking, she decided to confront Mark at his workplace. She begged him to stop his personal and legal attacks on her. The rest of the story brings us to the officer's statement that day outside of Angela's hospital room.

Is she a hardened criminal, to be despised? Is she fit to be re-integrated into society? Would the lens of her family physician, privy to her past and present, who sees the whole person, change that opinion? Hopefully.

20 Understanding the Whole Person without Knowing the Whole Person

Barbara Jones and Judith Belle Brown

When I first met Barney Gilchrist 10 years ago, he was not a happy man. His 55-year-old wife, Ramona, had recently died, and he'd moved from the city to the suburbs to start a new life with his 17-year-old son, Ian. He'd promised Ramona he would always take care of Ian, and his concern about high youth unemployment rates was only one of a long list of his anxieties. A slightly built and balding 60-year-old man, he arrived with a new complaint every couple of weeks and regaled me with tales of his woes.

Despite all these visits over many years, I never really found out much about Barney's past. At each visit Barney had new symptoms he wanted to discuss and consistently resisted my efforts to focus on the psychosocial issues I thought must be underlying his problems. Barney told me how devastated he was at the loss of his wife and implied that he'd been successful at his work, although he never revealed what that was. He explained he had retired early because of a heart problem and was now living comfortably on his savings. Barney, a sad man, was obviously lonely, although he would not admit as much. I did hear on occasion about the lady he had met during a trip abroad and how he had hopes that this relationship might flourish in the future.

I was struck by the fact that Barney appeared to have a need to impress me. He wanted me to believe he was a competent and well-liked man. To this day I don't know the origin of his "heart problem," given that in the 10 years I have known him, Barney has not shown any signs of heart disease. The reason for his early retirement I still don't know, but he did admit after a year or so that he was actually on a pension and did not have any savings. He apologized for deceiving me, although it was the least of my concerns. His stories about his lady friend also sounded like an effort to impress – perhaps to impress himself as well as his doctor.

As well as being lonely, Barney was bored. He had not managed to establish new friendships or interests in the community. Finally, after a couple of years, Barney agreed to talk about the activities he would like to become involved in. He said that he'd always wanted to take up lawn bowling. Lawn bowling is a common activity for older people in our country, and every suburb has a club. With a little prompting from me, he contacted the local club and returned to proudly tell me that he had become a member.

I did not see Barney much after that. He soon became too busy to fit in visits to the doctor. Within a year, he was treasurer of the club. Then the law changed to allow them to install gambling machines. On one of his rare visits, I asked how much money they were making from gambling and was staggered at his reply. They were building a new clubhouse and restaurant and still could not spend all the revenue from their "new enterprise." Barney now bounced in about once a year and couldn't wipe the smile off his face. His medical problems receded and didn't seem to trouble him at all. A far cry from the rather stooped and whining man I knew 10 years ago. And all because of lawn bowling.

Barney's story illuminates how much our interpersonal and contextual factors influence our experience of illness, and how much illness results purely from these factors as well. I have no doubt that the symptoms Barney presented to me so often early in our relationship were genuine. If he stopped to think about it now, Barney could probably discover some of those symptoms most days. But they no longer have the same meaning for him, and he no longer feels the need to seek medical assistance. It was not easy for me to resist Barney's attempts to medicalize his problems, which was a safer option for him rather than admitting he was not coping as well as he thought he should. Nor was it easy to help Barney to address his real problems. The easy route for both of us would have been to treat him as an invalid, but Barney would be in a very different situation today had we taken that course.

Barney's story also reminds us that we cannot solve our patients' problems for them. They must do that for themselves. But we can facilitate the process with minimal intervention. Who knows how long it would have taken Barney to make that first step of contacting a lawn bowling club on his own – a very scary first step for him. That's all I really did to help – just made that first step a little easier. All the rest Barney did for himself. I find it very reassuring that I don't have to do more than that. Sometimes it is difficult for doctors to find time to spend on their patients' psychosocial problems, but everyone can do as much as I did with Barney. And in the long run, it has saved me a lot of time in unnecessary visits for minor problems and also saved the health system unnecessary costs.

My experience with Barney illustrates the fact that we don't need to know everything about our patients in order to help them. It is often helpful to know more about their background and psyche. But it may not be necessary. Even after all this time I know very little about Barney. We need not necessarily despair about patients who are reluctant to tell us about themselves. Having said that, however, it was a watershed when Barney decided to trust me with the truth about himself. When he no longer had to waste energy on concealing the truth, it became easier to begin to address some of his real problems.

Barney's story also underscores the importance of the patient-doctor relationship. He needed someone to turn to in those early days. Barney needed someone who would accept him for himself and would be tolerant of his illness behavior and his fumbling attempts to establish a new life. Doctors are generally safe people to talk to, and we see many patients who are not really sick, but need someone to talk to. Often patients will take some time to establish whether they can trust us with their secrets. And we need to accept their right to try us out before they decide to trust us.

Barney touched my life as I touched his. I delight in seeing him come in now as a confident and happy man. I feel I had a small part to play in that happiness. Through knowing Barney I am reassured that we can help our patients make profound changes if we simply accept them as worthwhile human beings, listen to them, resist their attempts to establish unhealthy behavior patterns and support their efforts to make difficult but necessary changes in their lives. Even the busiest doctors can do that.

COMPONENT III

Finding Common Ground

Judith Belle Brown, Moira Stewart
and W. Wayne Weston

Finding common ground, the third interactive component of the patient-centered method, is the process through which the patient and doctor reach a mutual understanding and mutual agreement in three key areas: defining the problem, establishing the goals and priorities of treatment and/or management, and identifying the roles to be assumed by both the patient and the doctor. To reach common ground often requires that two potentially divergent viewpoints be brought together in a reasonable plan (Kon 2010; Edwards and Elwyn 2009). Once agreement is reached on the nature of the problems, the patient and doctor must determine the goals and priorities of treatment and/or management. What will be the patients' involvement in the treatment plan? Do the plans make sense in terms of the patients' perceptions of their health, their understanding of their disease and their unique illness experience? How well do the treatment plans match the values and preferences of the patient? Can the patient afford the medication, and can he or she cope with the demands of treatment? Finally, how do the parties involved – patients and doctors – define their roles in this interaction?

DEFINING THE PROBLEM

Seeking an understanding or explanation for worrisome physical or emotional symptoms is a fundamental human need. Most patients want a "name" or label for their disease to help them gain some sense of control over what is happening to them (Kleinman 1988; McWhinney 1989; Cassell 1991; Wood 1991; Helman 2007; Lang, Floyd and Beine 2000). When patients can assign a label to their problems it helps them understand the cause, what to expect in terms of the course or timeline of the problem and what the outcome will be (Cooper 1998). It also assists them in regaining some degree of mastery over what may have been a frightening symptom.

Patients have usually developed some ideas – their "explanatory model" (Kleinman 1988; Helman 2007) about their problem before presenting to the doctor. Failure to elicit the patient's perspective may jeopardize agreement on the nature of the problem(s). Without some common understanding about what is wrong, it is difficult for a patient and doctor to agree on a treatment protocol or plan of management that is acceptable to both. It is not essential that the physician share the same perspective on the problem as the patient, but the doctor's explanation and recommended treatment must at least be consistent with the patient's point of view and make sense in the patient's world.

In defining and describing the problem, it is essential that doctors give the information in language patients can understand, thus complex medical terms and clinical language should be avoided. If patients are intimidated by medical jargon, it may limit their ability to express their ideas and concerns or even to raise important questions. Failure to elicit these patients' expressions may result in a failure to find common ground. Patients need to be encouraged to ask questions and not fear being ridiculed or embarrassed for not knowing or not understanding technical terms and procedures. Just as active listening is key to exploring patients' illness experiences, it is also central to finding common ground. Thus it is important to understand and acknowledge patients' perspectives on their problems.

DEFINING THE GOALS

Once the patient and doctor have reached a mutual understanding and agreement about the problem, the next step is to explore the goals and priorities of treatment and/or the management plan. If doctors ignore their patient's expectations and ideas about treatment and/or management, they risk not understanding their patients, who may in turn become angry or hurt by this perceived lack of interest or concern. Some patients will become more demanding in a determined effort to be heard; others will become withdrawn and feel abandoned. Patients may be reluctant to listen to their doctors' treatment recommendations unless they feel that their ideas and opinions had first been heard and respected.

Timing is important. If the physician inquires about the patient's ideas about what is causing their problems too early in the interview, the patient may think that the doctor doesn't know what is going on. On the other hand, if the doctor waits until the end of the consultation, time may be wasted on issues irrelevant to the patient. The process of finding common ground begins right from the start of the interview by eliciting the patient's full list of concerns and showing respect for their ideas and questions. Doctors need to actively engage their patients and explicitly inquire about their expectations. For example, a physician might say, "Can you help me to understand what we might do together to get your diabetes under control?" Often it is helpful to pick up on patients' cues that hint at their feelings, ideas or expectations. For example, a patient may express frustration about the failure of treatment recommendations to help: "I have had this back pain for three weeks now and none of the pain medication you gave me has helped. I just can't bear the pain!" The doctor should avoid becoming defensive in trying to justify previous recommendations. Instead, it is more helpful to address the patient's frustration and the implied message that something must be done: "You sound fed up with the length of time this pain has dragged on and would like a different approach to treatment."

Often patients find it awkward or difficult to provide suggestions about their health goals or the treatment or management of their diseases. Some patients may feel that their opinion lacks validity and value, while others may defer to the authority of the "expert" clinician in the decision-making process. Physicians need to encourage patients' participation with statements such as: "I'm really interested in your point of view, especially since you are the one who has to live with our decision about these treatments." It is important for doctors to clearly explain the treatment and/or management options and to engage patients in a mutual discussion of the pros and cons of different approaches. It is also important to acknowledge and address the patients' questions and concerns so that patients feel heard and understood. In clarifying patients' agreement with a specific plan, questions such as the following can be very useful: "Can you think of any difficulties in following through on this?" "Is there anything we can do to make this treatment plan easier for you?" "Do you need more time to think this over?" "Is there anybody you would like to talk to about this treatment?" These questions and others help forge partnerships with patients; they are, as Tuckett *et al.* (1985) described, "meetings between experts" – the physician is the expert in the biomedical basis of the problems, but the patient is the expert in how the problems are affecting him and how options for treatment mesh with his values, preferences and personal situation.

Establishing the goals of treatment and/or management must also take into account the expectations and feelings of physicians. Sometimes doctors are concerned that patients may ask for something they disagree with, because they are not comfortable with confrontation and with saying no. As a result they may prefer to avoid the issue, but then finding common ground will not be achieved. Doctors can become frustrated and disheartened when patients are not concordant with treatment protocols and management plans. But what physicians call "non-compliance" may be the patient's expressions of disagreement about treatment goals. As Quill and Brody (1996) observe: "Final choices belong to patients, but these choices gain meaning, richness, and accuracy if they are the result of a process of mutual influence and understanding between physician and patient" (p. 765).

DEFINING THE ROLES OF PATIENT AND DOCTOR

Inherent in articulating the roles to be assumed by the patient and doctor is a definition of mutual responsibility for the actions that will follow. These may be quite simple, such as: "How about I see you again in one month to check that this new medication is lowering your blood pressure." Implicit in this statement is the patient's agreement to use the medication as prescribed, and the doctor's desire for future follow-up. Certain situations, however, may be more complex and therefore require an explicit statement of the roles to be assumed by the patient and the doctor.

Sometimes there is strong disagreement about the nature of the problem or the goals and priorities for treatment. When such an impasse occurs, it is important to look at the relationship between the patient and the doctor, and at their perception of each other's roles. Doctors, for example, when caring for a cancer patient, may see themselves as wanting to bring about remission, and may expect the patient to assume the role of a passive recipient of treatment. Patients, however, may be seeking a physician who expresses concern and interest in their well-being, and who is prepared to treat them in the least invasive manner, viewing them as autonomous individuals with a right to have a voice in deciding among various forms of treatment. This is not such a dilemma for doctors when the various forms of treatment are equally effective, but physicians are understandably concerned when the patient chooses a treatment that they consider either less efficacious or even harmful.

Finding common ground about a patient's role in the decision-making process does not necessarily imply that the patient will assume an active role. Patients' levels of participation in decision-making may fluctuate depending on their emotional and physical capabilities. Thus doctors need to be flexible and responsive to potential changes in their patients' involvement. Some patients may be too sick or too overwhelmed by the burden of their illness to actively participate in their care. Others may find decisions about treatment options too complex and confusing, hence delegating the decision-making to the clinician.

THE PROCESS OF FINDING COMMON GROUND

In the process of finding common ground, it is the doctor's responsibility to define and describe the problem. This may be as clear-cut, such as "you have a strep throat," or ultimately more complex and uncertain, such as "there are several possibilities to explain your symptoms, so what I suggest we do is …" Next it is important to provide the patient with an opportunity to ask questions. This is not simply an "okay?", but an intentional engagement of the patient: "What do *you* think?" Some patients may retort with, "I don't know? You are the doctor!" Doctors need to respond with a comment such as: "Yes, and I will provide you with information and my opinion, but your ideas and wishes are important in making our plan together." This is when information sharing begins.

The patient and doctor can then participate in a mutual discussion of their shared understanding of the problem and how it can best be addressed. At the conclusion of their discussion of treatment options and management goals it is the clinician's responsibility to explicitly clarify the patient's understanding and agreement. It is during this summation that the doctor and patient can make specific their respective roles in achieving the mutually agreed upon treatment goals. This may be as simple as agreeing on how follow-up plans will be arranged, or as complex as a discussion of how a cancer patient in the palliative phase needs the doctor to assume a caring role versus a curative stance.

CONCLUSION

Finding common ground requires that patients and physicians reach a mutual understanding and mutual agreement on the nature of the problems, the goals and priorities of treatment and/or management, and their respective roles. Sometimes patients and doctors have divergent views in each of these areas. The process of finding a satisfactory resolution is not one of bargaining or negotiating but rather of moving towards a meeting of minds or finding common ground.

Preview of the Narratives

In this section, the narratives emphasize how the third component, finding common ground, can be the lynchpin of the patient-centered clinical method, but this is not without its challenges.

In the first narrative, **Chapter 21**, we witness the challenges in caring for people who are homeless. In this story we learn how the patient has experienced much trauma and violence in her life, yet she is a survivor.

She then faces an extremely serious medical condition that is potentially life-threatening. The patient is paralyzed with fear - the prospect of invasive surgery is untenable. Gently the physician seeks to build a relationship with a patient who avoids authority figures. With a tentative bond established, the crisis is averted, and they find common ground regarding the needed surgery. But this is just the beginning of the story, and finding common ground is ongoing between the patient and doctor as they circumvent the patient's many crises.

Chapter 22 demonstrates how attentive listening, an active presence, and communication all play a pivotal role in gaining trust – trust that is necessary for an effective patient-doctor relationship. It also highlights the critical distinction between the diagnosis of disease and the illness experience of patients, and how some patients need this explicitly clarified through effective communication to foster healing.

The next story, **Chapter 23**, emphasizes the role families play in finding common ground during acute illnesses and resuscitation. It illuminates the value of including families during the resuscitation process in order to foster healing and closure. Furthermore, it emphasizes how physicians can overcome institutional blindness to appreciate the suffering patient as a previously normal, functioning, non-sick individual – a mother, a wife, a gardener – a whole person.

When do we feel justified to act against the wishes of a patient in order to maintain his or her safety and forfeit finding common ground? **Chapter 24** reveals the struggles experienced by a physician who strives to build a trusting patient-doctor relationship with a woman who has both physical and social challenges. The goal is to provide her with a safe environment and preserve her dignity, but in the end they fail to find common ground, and the relationship is shattered. While this narrative may sound desolate, it offers many valuable lessons about being patient-centered.

We often think about finding common ground with patients as being focused on management or the treatment of a specific disease, often with a cure in mind. However, finding common ground can also be directly applied to how we help patients face a terminal disease and their decision about how they die. The two-part story in **Chapter 25** and **Chapter 26** serves as an illustration.

Chapter 27 exemplifies how relinquishing control on the part of both the physician and parent can be empowering in a patient's life. It also demonstrates how this behavior can facilitate finding common ground and can foster a solid foundation for a healthy, long-term patient-physician-family relationship.

Sometimes finding common ground is a precarious process that can easily unravel when patient's expectations and concerns remain unheard. **Chapter 28** underscores how the strength of the patient-doctor relationship preserves this pivotal component. Indeed, it is the patient's courage to address her dissatisfaction and the physician's ability to listen to the criticisms that lead them to successfully finding common ground.

Chapter 29 demonstrates how finding common ground can sometimes be a fine balance. In this story, the elderly patient's physical and emotional pain are tightly interwoven, reflecting a lifetime of loss and sorrow. This presents the physician with a monumental task in trying to relieve her patient's profound suffering. At times this feels overwhelming, yet the doctor perseveres in her attempts to alleviate her patient's multiple concerns. With time and constancy they strike a balance – the pain remains but becomes less of a burden for both the patient and the doctor.

We end this section with a story **Chapter 30** that examines the challenges of an adolescent with a long history of living with cancer and pain management. His story portrays the potentially fragile nature of the patient-doctor relationship and as such serves as a transition to the next section of this book, the foundation of patient-centered care – the patient-doctor relationship.

Narratives Illustrating Component III:
Finding Common Ground

21 Let It Be

Susan Woolhouse

Dr. Patel reflected on the visit she had just completed with her patient, Maddie. Reception had alerted her earlier in the morning that Maddie had dropped in, demanding, "I need to see Dr. Patel! It is very important!"

Dr. Patel had sighed – Maddie rarely seemed to visit the drop-in clinic – a clinic designed to make it easier for marginalized women like Maddie to access primary health care. Rather, Maddie would always appear, unannounced, during regular office hours. "Well, at least she is here," Dr. Patel thought, thankfully.

Dr. Patel strolled out to the waiting room and called Maddie's name. In a loud and gruff manner Maddie shouted in response, "What took you so long? I've been waiting *forever!*"

Without missing a beat, Dr. Patel replied, "It's nice to see you too. Glad to see you're in such a good mood!" Dr. Patel chuckled as she remembered Maddie's reaction to her own light-hearted sarcasm.

Maddie stood up, grinned and let out a hearty belly laugh. "I hope you had a good vacation. I thought you would want to see me and check my blood pressure. I know you've missed me!"

They both laughed as they walked into Dr. Patel' exam room. As Dr. Patel checked her blood pressure, Maddie inquired about her vacation. Turning the conversation back on Maddie, Dr. Patel asked, "So overall, how are you doing, Maddie?"

"Me?" she replied. "I'm doing okay, doc. But right now I gotta go. I don't have any more time to talk. Don't worry. I'll see you next week." With that, Maddie shuffled out the door.

Visits with Maddie weren't always so easy. In fact, Dr. Patel recalled a time when Maddie, a 57-year-old woman with multiple physical and mental health problems, had a temper tantrum in the hallway outside her office. She had screamed that she hated Dr. Patel and that no one was helping her. Dr. Patel, at her wit's end and frustrated with Maddie's escalating and very challenging behaviors, had firmly said to Maddie, "You can either act like an adult or a child. If you choose to continue to act like a child, I am leaving. Take your pick." Luckily, that hard-line approach worked, and a productive visit had followed. It took a few years for Dr. Patel to figure out how best to handle Maddie's roller-coaster moods and emotional dys-regulation. Similarly, it had taken just as long for Maddie to figure out how to work with Dr. Patel!

Maddie's life had been hard – a life filled with trauma, violence, and more recently, some very serious physical health problems. When Maddie and Dr. Patel first met, Maddie was living under a bridge and was extremely isolated. It was when Maddie reached rock-bottom that she and Dr. Patel had their first contact. When Maddie had experienced increasing problems with her coordination and balance, she had sought out relief for her symptoms at the local emergency room. Brain imaging had shown a large, unruptured cerebral aneurysm. The attending neurosurgeon wanted to admit Maddie immediately and operate. It was a matter of life or death. Maddie was over-whelmed and terrified. She fled the hospital.

Luckily, Maddie was connected to a program for homeless women at the clinic where Dr. Patel worked. When the staff heard of the gravity of Mad-die's situation, they had urged her to return to the hospital. Maddie had flatly refused. As the physician affiliated with the women's program, the team was hopeful that Dr. Patel could try and connect with Maddie next time she came to the clinic.

Because women like Maddie have such difficulties trusting others, espe-cially people in authority positions like physicians, Dr. Patel had known she would need help from other team members to make the first connec-tion. Here at the clinic, unlike a regular family practice, the engagement of marginalized women like Maddie often happened through a social service provider. The strong relationships that women attending this program had formed with the other staff allowed Dr. Patel to build trust vicariously.

The following week, Maddie arrived at the drop-in clinic. A staff member with whom Maddie had developed a positive relationship introduced her to Dr. Patel. Dr. Patel recalled that when she first saw Maddie, she had been sit-ting alone in a corner eating a snack. Dr. Patel had sat down and said gently, "Hi Maddie. My name is Dr. Patel and I am the doctor connected to the program. I hear you don't like doctors very much. I don't blame you one bit. I also hear that you've had a pretty tough time this last week. I'd like to help you."

Maddie had looked at Dr. Patel with tears running down her face, "I can't do this. I just can't. I won't go back to the hospital. I don't want to die."

Dr. Patel remembered saying, "This must be really scary. Why don't we spend a bit of time talking about what you feel you can do." This provided Dr. Patel with the opportunity to connect with Maddie and support her to get the medical care she so desperately needed.

With patience, perseverance and a bit of creativity, the team supported Maddie in returning to the hospital and having surgery. Dr. Patel visited Maddie in the hospital the day after the surgery. Although Maddie had been groggy and hooked up to many tubes, Maddie had grinned at Dr. Patel and said, "I did it, didn't I?"

It was in that moment that Dr. Patel had realized that she had passed the test. She had earned Maddie's trust. The patient-doctor relationship was solidified. She had also learned what an amazingly strong women Maddie was. Maddie had been able to face a terrifying surgical procedure with humor and grace.

Although Maddie's life stabilized after the surgery – she found housing, began to take her medications faithfully and had the support of a case manager – she still struggled. Maddie suffered from chronic obstructive pulmonary disease (COPD) and cirrhosis, both of which were progressing. She was short of breath at rest and had been admitted to the hospital for an episode of hepatic encephalopathy. Her coping skills were minimal and her insight was poor, making discussions with Maddie about her prognosis difficult for Dr. Patel, as she was never quite sure if Maddie truly understood the gravity of her situation. What was clear was that talking too much about her situation only caused Maddie more distress.

Maybe that morning's visit hadn't accomplished much medically. In fact, it looked like Dr. Patel hadn't accomplished much of anything. But that visit had been very important. Dr. Patel recalled a presentation at a conference characterizing four types of clinical encounters: routine, ceremony, drama and routine drama. "Routine" visits were characterized by brevity and use of a biomedical model. "Ceremonies" often used rituals such as vitamin B12 injections for addressing chronic pain. "Dramas," on the other hand, were characterized by emotional intensity and psychosocial complexity, such as when a physician has to deliver bad news. Lastly, "routine dramas" were similar to "routine" encounters in that they were brief and frequent; however, they were also driven by constant and repetitive crises that often went unresolved. Dr. Patel's first visit with Maddie was most like a drama. Their subsequent visits consisted primarily of "routine dramas."

After reflecting on the last visit, Dr. Patel recognized the ceremonial nature of these encounters. The ritual of taking Maddie's blood pressure and simply "checking in" had become an important function in Maddie's life – it validated her fears and anxieties. It also reassured her that someone cared and would be there for her at the end of her life. Dr. Patel stopped trying to get Maddie to understand just how serious things were. Finding common ground with Maddie had become simply allowing her to just be.

As Maddie had shuffled out the door that morning, Dr. Patel had said goodbye and agreed that they touch base the following week, "Just to see how your blood pressure is doing."

22 The Alliance

Sofian Al-Samak, Tanya Thornton and Judith Belle Brown

"There must be something wrong!" Franco insisted. "Doc, I've got chest pain, I can't breathe, I'm going to die, I can feel it!" he shouted, starting to tremble. Franco paused to inhale a deep breath of oxygen from the mask adherent to his face, which fortunately muffled out the volume of his panicked outbursts.

Dr. Purcell, the ER physician, inhaled slowly and sighed, trying to calm his inner frustrations. "Mr. Miller, we have checked your heart, the tests are all negative, we should –"

"You must have missed something, check again!" Franco barked. "You're not hearing me! I want to call my father!" he ordered, believing he needed an advocate.

"No problem," Dr. Purcell replied, heading for the door, thankful he could finally escape this uncomfortable encounter.

As he walked towards the nursing station, he reviewed the details of Mr. Miller's presentation: 25-year-old male, central chest pain of two hours duration associated with arm paresthesias and shortness of breath … similar episodes in the remote past; episodes becoming more frequent of late. His cardiac enzymes were repeated and returned negative – *this was not a heart attack*, Dr. Purcell assured himself. Mr. Miller's chest X-ray was normal, his electrocardiogram was normal, and additional blood work to rule out other conditions with similar symptoms was pristine.

His deliberation was interrupted by a commotion coming from Franco's room. Upon entering, Dr. Purcell found Franco pacing the length of the stretcher.

"You need to give him something to calm him down," the nurse beseeched, "and his father wants to talk to you," she added, handing Dr. Purcell the phone.

"Ok, give him some valium," he ordered, while writing the dose on the chart and balancing the phone on his shoulder. From the other end, a male voice began berating accusations and threatening litigation for the inadequate and inappropriate care of his son Franco. Dr. Purcell, losing patience, hung up and stormed out of Franco's room.

Security guards appeared at Franco's door. Franco stopped pacing. He started to cry. "I just want help, I need to get well," he sobbed. He was discharged, escorted from the department and advised to return if things changed or worsened.

Despite consulting his family physician and investigations in the ER being negative, Franco was never reassured. "No doctor really knows what's going on with me," he explained to the physician on his subsequent ER visit. "I'm so frustrated, I can't understand why I have pain if it's not my heart. I can't stand not knowing what's going on, why I feel this way. I can't sleep at night now that my pain is getting worse. I'm so worried." The ER doctor charted in the diagnosis box: "chest pain nyd" – denoting chest pain not yet diagnosed, meaning: not classifiable based on current diagnostic criteria. What it should read is "patient suffering not fully understood." The ER physician threw the chart in the pile to be signed off and moved on to the next patient.

It was late on a Friday night when Franco returned again to the ER. He was plagued by fears of having a sinister disease that doctors couldn't diagnose. Since his last visit, he had not returned to work as a laborer in a furniture store, thinking the physical exertion might strain his heart. Likewise, he ceased his daily jog. At home, as tensions mounted; he and his girlfriend began arguing. Furthermore, without his minimum-wage income, Franco was no longer able to assist his mother financially, and as an only child, this was painfully burdensome. Franco felt guilty and useless. Concurrently, his chest pain episodes became more frequent and disabling.

That Friday night, Dr. Johnston was starting her third back-to-back night shift. As she trudged over to the nursing desk, already fatigued, the nurse slapped a chart in her hand, "Good luck with this frequent flyer," she smirked. Dr. Johnston never liked that term – frequent flyer. Although it simply referred to someone who repeatedly returned seeking care from the ER, it conveyed a negative, attention-seeking undertone. Dr. Johnston looked down at the chief complaint, printed in caps at the top of the chart: CHEST PAIN.

The nurse called over her shoulder, "I put his old chart on the desk for you." Dr. Johnston glanced over at a voluminous file folder, its papers askew. She glanced up at the rack of pending patients to be seen: empty. Her heart became lighter, "*Okay, let's see what's been done for this gentleman,*" she thought, ready to tackle the tome before her. As she digested the facts, she realized that Franco had previously had every appropriate investigation done over the past few months to ensure there was nothing life-threatening occurring within his body. His heart, lungs and gastrointestinal tract had been probed, poked and peered into. Nothing appeared abnormal, nor could the tests to date explain his symptoms. She read how he had called his father as an advocate, but that had escalated the already strained situation. Previous physicians felt unsafe in his agitated presence. He became verbally abusive. Dr. Johnston paused. "*Why is he convinced he is sick?*" she wondered. She strode into his room, determined to get to the bottom of things once and for all. Dr. Johnston pulled up a stool and sat down parallel to Franco's bed. His hair was greasy, and his eyes fatigued, but he shook her hand with strength and forced a smile upon introductions. "Franco, I've read your chart, but I want to hear what's going on in your own words. Why are you convinced that your chest pain is from your heart?"

"Well, doesn't it usually indicate a heart attack?" Franco asked.

"Not always, sometimes it can feel like a heart attack, but can be the result of the mind's response to stress," Dr. Johnston paused, giving him time to digest this. "How are things at home?" she cautiously inquired.

"You're the first doctor to ask me that," Franco replied. "I'm afraid. The fear of not knowing what's causing the pain has taken over my whole life. I'm not the same person I was a year ago. I need to get better. My mom and girlfriend are relying on me. My dad is working out of the country; I'm the only one they have."

"How long have you had the increased responsibility of caring for your mom?" Dr. Johnston asked.

"For the last four months," Franco admitted. "What if –"

"Just a minute," Dr. Johnston interjected. Although not usually wanting to interrupt a patient, she didn't want him to get worked up, and so she probed on in a different direction. "I realize you have 'what if' concerns … what-if you never get well again – I've read your chart … but 'what if' I could help you get better?"

Franco looked up from the bed. His voice quivered, "Really, you can?"

"Well, let's review what's been done." Dr. Johnston walked him through step-by-step investigations and clarified how a physician rules out diseases. She explained, "You've had all the tests necessary to confidently exclude a heart attack and other life-threatening conditions." Dr. Johnston itemized the tests and what they ruled out and why she could, with assurance, confirm the absence of organic pathology as the source of his chest pain. "What we haven't excluded yet is a diagnosis of panic attacks," Dr. Johnston suggested. Worried he may become defensive, she continued on, "These can cause as much chest pain and fear of death as a heart attack, but the good news is there is treatment for this and you can continue working and jogging and helping your mom."

The first tentative smile emerged. "I never thought of panic attacks, but it makes sense, my mom has them all the time."

Dr. Johnston remained in the room, seated at his bedside for another 30 minutes. It was so quiet in his room that the nurse came to check on

Dr. Johnston's safety, only to find the two absorbed in conversation, appearing as friends and allies. Indeed, an alliance had formed, and together they were devising a management plan.

Dr. Johnston had perceived Franco's anxiety but couldn't understand it. Instead of ignoring this incongruence, she explored it, without preconceived notions. She attentively listened to Franco's symptoms, validated his concerns, respected and addressed his fears and en route, gained his trust. He valued understanding the process of diagnosis and how physicians could confidently rule out diseases he was worried about. This time, he was reassured. He had been heard and he could now hear the physician's advice for treatment. Previous physicians had focused on ruling out diseases, without attempting to heal his suffering through communication. The faith he had lost in his care and his health care providers was slowly being restored by Dr. Johnston's meticulous explanations. It was a mutually satisfying visit, and the last one for Franco for a very long time.

23 Infusing Humanity into the Resuscitative Context

Tanya Thornton and Judith Belle Brown

"Oh don't worry, doctor. Jane, my youngest daughter, will be here shortly to answer your questions," Edna reassured. As she tried to get comfortable lying on the stretcher of our busy rural emergency department, her face furrowed again, and she paled.

"The pain is back?"I asked, already knowing the answer.

"Only when I move now, doctor, it comes in the middle of my back," she exhaled as she settled in one position, her facial color returning momentarily. "Could I have something for the pain?"

I rechecked her latest vitals on the monitor. Her blood pressure was still too low to give her any effective narcotic pain medicine due to the risk of making her threateningly hypotensive. "In a few minutes," I reassured. *Where is the nurse? She was supposed to put in a second intravenous for fluids to bring up Edna's blood pressure.* "I'll be right back, I'm going to look at your chest X-ray," I said, rushing off. As I passed by the nursing station, I called over my shoulder, "Page me when her daughter arrives, I need to talk to her."

I plopped myself down in the quiet X-ray viewing area. Finally, silence. I flicked on the view box light – a quiet hum and bright light interrupted the peaceful rest. I slapped up the chest X-ray.

Edna had been brought in an hour ago by paramedics with "sudden onset of back pain at rest," which had resolved en route in the ambulance. When I spoke with her on initial presentation in the ER, she recounted her story with energy. She lived on her own, but her two daughters kept a "close eye" on her, she explained. "Thoracic aneurysm repaired four months ago, been feeling well since," Edna narrated. Smiling as she continued chatting, Edna shared what a valuable source of help her daughters had been during her long ICU stay. Although she did not like to bother them, she was relieved that her daughter Jane would be here soon to answer my questions.

I looked up at the view box – my own heart started to race: "*Oh no!*" I stared, defying myself to comprehend what I saw: a massively widened mediastinum – indicating a ruptured thoracic aneurysm. The cause of her back pain was a tear in the major artery carrying blood from the heart to the rest of the body – the artery that Edna told me she had repaired four months earlier! *How could this be?* As I started to rise from the view box, I heard the overhead page: "Code blue, resusc 1, code blue, resusc 1." I ran.

When I arrived in the resuscitation room, there was a flurry of activity. One nurse was bagging Edna, while another one was doing chest compressions. An unfamiliar face was in the corner of the room – it was Jane. "Please do all you can," she begged.

"We will," I assured her, not making eye contact. My attention was distracted by sequences of code protocols, the frenetic activity of people accumulating in the room and the realization of the inevitable terminality of Edna's condition. After intubation, I looked up to see that Jane had left the room. I quickly asked the nurse to see if Jane wanted to be present for the resuscitation. The nurse who had been recording the sequence of events and medications looked up with raised eyebrows. "Thank you," I said, indicating yes, she had indeed heard me correctly. Within a few minutes, the patient's daughter returned. "Thanks, I thought I had to leave," Jane said, straining a smile.

I explained what had happened – her mother's thoracic aneurysm had likely ruptured. I described along the way what we had done in a resuscitation attempt. Jane moved closer to her mother's feet, touched them lightly, and nodded. "Do all you can," she whispered. I returned to the algorithm we follow for code protocols, dictating orders while ever cognizant of Jane's presence.

"Is your sister coming too?" I asked. Jane was impressed I knew she had a sister. I added, "Your mother couldn't stop talking about you two and what a wonderful gift you were after her surgery."

"No, she's not in town," Jane said. She paused, then asked, "Can I call her? Maybe mom would recognize her voice." Although they say hearing is the last sense to go during the death process, I knew that Edna's hearing was all but gone now. *Nevertheless, what would it hurt?* "Sure," I replied. The nurse again raised her eyebrows. I dialed the number, the nurses continued bagging and doing chest compressions. Jane held the phone to her mother's ear so that her sister could say goodbye.

Meanwhile, the heart monitor hummed its slow, infrequent pitch, signaling a non-life sustaining rhythm. Edna's skin had mottled, her eyes had glazed over without recognition of our presence. I realized that this dynamic 82-year-old woman, whom an hour earlier had told me in an animated fashion about her passion for gardening, was no longer with us.

We "ran the code" as Jane watched the entire process, with myself and the nurses explaining along the way. Suddenly, I was aware of how to word my orders, my out-loud thinking. Jane's presence required me to consider the callousness of the words I chose, and I am a better physician for it. It enabled me to connect with her, gain her trust and find common ground, when a decision regarding resuscitation cessation was required.

Amidst the beeps and my racing thoughts of resuscitation code protocols, I realized that Jane had hung up the phone. She was again observing reflectively from the end of the stretcher. She moved closer and stroked her mom's cool cheek, then cupped her even colder hand ever so gently. She leaned over and whispered, "I love you mom." Then Jane looked up and said in a quiet but assured voice, "It's okay, you can stop now. Thank you." This was the most comforting moment I had ever experienced during a resuscitation attempt. The weight of the tasks at hand, the responsibility of the decisions, and the burden of having to share with family the outcome of an "unsuccessful code" suddenly lifted. The frantic activity minutes before was replaced with a healing calmness in the room – an awareness of mutual closure that was instantly healing for both daughter and physician.

In retrospect, the phone conversation had given Jane moments to reflect on the type of life her mother had led and what her mother would have wanted in this situation, given the probable poor outcome. Through open communication, with a presence at the resuscitative bedside, and with trust rapidly building the bonds of this new family-patient-physician relationship, Jane was able to choose the way she wanted to say goodbye.

Although I saw Edna as an elderly terminal patient with mottled skin and fixed, dilated pupils, and although I stood there calculating the duration of time without cerebral blood flow, realizing her inevitable death, I also knew her as a person and as a mother. She had white hair, a wedding ring, and well-manicured nails. Would I have recalled these details had I not considered her humanness? Would I have appreciated her as a person if I had not invited her daughter to be present? I don't know. What I do believe is that the experience changed me as a physician and as a person. It has imbued me with a sense of personal and professional satisfaction.

In stressful, acute circumstances, our reliance on technology and the sterilization of the trauma room from family can be used as armor, protecting physicians and nurses from deeper and more challenging realities of practice – the patient-centered aspects of care inherent to sudden acute illnesses, suffering and death.

However, the dehumanization of the resuscitation process can be avoided through actions, which reflect respect for patients as people. The resuscitation team is then seen as caring for the patient, rather than carrying out a process or "running a code". The process can be infused with a humanness and sensitivity reflective of patient-centered end-of-life care. In the high-tech environment of the resuscitation room, connecting with others can be healing for the patient and family, as well as for the nurses and physicians caring for them.

24 A Tale of Spunk and Smoke

Susan Woolhouse and Judith Belle Brown

Helen was a patient about whom I was warned. Colleagues had told me so many stories about her that I wasn't expecting us to get along. But it didn't take me long to admire this strong-willed woman. Helen was full of spunk. She was a no-nonsense woman who didn't beat around the bush. She had a similar expectation of me. "Just get to the point," Helen would tell me as my earnest explanations took lengthy and tangential turns. There was never any worry that you didn't know what Helen was thinking. She was forthright – using language that would set your hair on fire.

I first met 51-year-old Helen after receiving a phone call from the nurse who worked at our satellite clinic. This clinic provided health and social services to people living in an attached supportive housing unit. Helen had been there for 18 months and had been using our services intermittently during that time. I was being asked to assess some burns she had received to her ear and neck after accidentally setting her hair on fire while smoking a cigarette.

When I reached Helen's apartment I was met by the strong smell of nicotine. Helen was smoking when I entered the room and introduced myself. Disheveled, with missed button holes on her shirt, her shoelaces untied, and with food stains on her skirt, Helen held her head up high, put her hand out and introduced herself with confidence. Her arm waved grandly with her choreiform movements, and her words were hard to understand. There was a huge burn oozing with pus on the side of her head. I managed to catch her hand, and we held on to one another with a firm grip, staring at each other in the eyes. I think she was daring me to look away. But, I didn't look away. "It's lovely to meet you Helen," I said. She smirked.

Helen had been formally diagnosed with Huntington's disease two years ago, but she didn't need to have doctors tell her this. She knew the symptoms all too well. As Helen told me in one of our later visits: "My mom died like an animal in one of those jails they call a nursing home," and her sister was nearing a similar fate. Dying in a nursing home terrified Helen. "Over my dead body. I won't go to one of those places. No way!" Helen announced with steely determination.

Helen not only posed a safety hazard to herself but to others in her building. She was likely to burn the building down with her unsafe smoking habits. The landlord had given her an eviction notice. Helen was fast on her way to becoming homeless. The health care team involved in Helen's care had a month to think of other possible solutions before her eviction date. Unfortunately, it was the middle of winter, and it was cold outside.

Helen could not manage on her own. Although she was aware of this, she was too proud to admit it to anyone. So, she coped by being creative and resourceful. Helen often offered shelter to others in exchange for help with activities of daily living. This often put Helen in unsafe positions, but she felt the benefits of this independence outweighed any risk of harm.

Understanding the proximal and distal contexts of Helen's life allowed me to better understand her struggles and her choices. Clearly, Helen's biggest fear was losing her independence. She had lost control over her physical body (her bowels, bladder and many voluntary movements) and was holding onto her "marbles" with every ounce of energy she could muster. As Helen put it, "I will not wait until I go nuts" – alluding to the inevitable dementia and psychiatric sequelae of Huntington's.

With this increasing understanding of Helen's situation, I began to realize the comfort that Helen derived from our visits in the quiet safety of my office. Sometimes we would just sit in silence – silence that was eventually interrupted by Helen's patience being tested: "Aren't you going to say something?" Trust with Helen was hard-earned but helped to establish the early phases of our relationship. I reminded myself that trusting someone can make them feel more vulnerable and open to being hurt.

As we got to know one another better, I felt that there was increased trust between the two of us. I asked more personal questions, and Helen spoke more about her past. I began to appreciate just how challenging it had been for her to watch her mother's health fail and to witness her mother become more and more dependent on Helen and her father. "She had lost all her pride at the end," Helen told me. Despite this increase in trust, our relationship was always tenuous.

Helen was becoming increasingly stubborn – she was refusing any assistance from home care and the Huntington's society. In fact, she refused almost all assistance. Pride can have its price. My concern revolved around Helen's increasingly volatile mood and poor memory. At our last visit, she could not remember the date and had forgotten my name. She was also not wearing clothes appropriate to the cold weather outside. Although her mini-mental status exam was 20/25, I was quite concerned that her disease, in addition to her personality, was interfering with her judgment and poor insight. Helen refused a psychiatric assessment, making it difficult to elucidate just what level of neurocognitive impairment she was suffering.

The situation culminated into a crisis when Helen left her supportive housing unit as her eviction day was fast approaching. She decided that she was better off without any of us and "our talk of nursing homes." "I'd be better off dead in a snow bank!" she shouted to staff as she walked out the door of her apartment building. Into the cold, wintery day she went, with only a rusty shopping cart and a sleeping bag. She had no money. We assumed that she had gone off to her usual hang-out, a local homeless drop-in. It was cold enough outside that if Helen did not find a safe indoor place, she was at risk of dying.

I made the difficult decision to certify her under the Mental Health Act, ultimately forcing Helen to get a psychiatric assessment, even if it was against her will. I needed a second opinion. I tried to convince myself that my intentions were ultimately in her best interests and not self-indulgent.

It was one of those miserable moments as a physician. As soon as she saw me she started swearing and swatting at me. The police had to block the doors to prevent her from leaving and then she simply collapsed and sat on the floor. It was a difficult and heart-wrenching situation. Helen had trusted me and I felt like I had betrayed her. The patient-doctor relationship that had taken so long to build had shattered in a matter of moments. She looked bewildered and hurt. Helen was taken to the hospital, assessed as "competent" and discharged back to the streets. Helen refused to see me or any other members of her health care team again.

The subtle and complex behavioral changes in Huntington's disease made assessment and management of Helen difficult. What part was Helen's innate personality, and what part was the disease? Could the two really be separated, and was her behavior clinically relevant? I struggled with the issue of Helen's ability to understand and to appreciate her situation fully. Although she was found competent, Helen had many symptoms consistent with cognitive decline. Even if she did have early dementia, did I have the right to act against her wishes?

Do I regret certifying Helen? I don't think so. I do regret that it happened in a way that made her feel demeaned and disempowered. Those are moments we don't forget as physicians. I am not sure how it could have happened differently though. The line between individual autonomy and protection of life is murky at best. Are these concepts as irreconcilable as they feel? Physicians struggle to minimize the influence of their power in their relationships with patients. However, as Helen reminds us, our power can feel overwhelming and subsume the relationship.

Many feelings arise when I think about Helen. Above all, I have admiration for her. While suffering from a horrible illness, she was able to maintain a fierce pride. She had a strong will to live – just on her terms.

25 Indelible Ink – Part 1

**Dori Seccareccia, Judith Belle Brown
and Tanya Thornton**

Oona's mark on my memory was made with indelible ink. She taught me more about the meaning of palliative care than any textbook or lecture ever could. This is her story.

Oona and her husband were skeptical of traditional medicine and were using alternative therapies to treat her cancer. Her pain had become so severe that she was willing to be admitted for an assessment, even though she distrusted hospitals and was leery of physicians.

I liked her immediately despite the prophecy of her being a "difficult" patient. We connected. She was a beautiful woman who emitted rays of spirit and courage. As she told her story, her soft-spoken words could not hide her will and determination, as well as the accompanying pain and suffering.

Vestiges of the initial shock of the diagnosis were still palpable. "I was only 48 years old when I was told I had colon cancer … only 48! I exercised every day, I ate well, I have never smoked, and I don't drink. How could I have cancer?" She paused before continuing on, "I love teaching, I miss the students – they need me and I need them. It isn't fair."

She began to weep, then stopped abruptly when Carlos, her husband, interjected, "Come on Oona, you know we're going to beat this. Look how far you've come – two years already, we're winning! You've got to win – for Jessica and Brent, they're only teenagers – and for us."

Oona was a teacher, a mom and a wife. She was a woman who had everything to live for and nothing to lose in fighting to keep it all. She was on a mission to get her pain under control; she saw this as the means to regain control of her life. The ferocious independence emanating from her eyes made me believe that Oona just might overcome the odds.

Oona had valid reasons to be upset and untrusting of the medical world. When she was first diagnosed, she was showered with support and the hope of a cure. What they were saying was exactly what Oona was hoping to hear. She had surgery and subsequent chemotherapy. The chemotherapy took its toll, but "it was worth it to get rid of the alien in my body," Oona asserted. The next year was good, until she thought she was gaining weight. Although she looked seven months pregnant, it was not the miracle of life growing within her, but the cancer. There was no further surgery to be offered, and chemotherapy was no longer aimed at a cure, but at *palliation*! Oona was devastated.

Despite three surgeons telling her that the mass was inoperable and that there was no cure available, Oona remained certain that after we got her pain under control, and after her herbalist "shrunk the tumor," she would find someone to "cut out the monster." Although Oona spoke in a determined fashion, I was sure I could hear a whisper of doubt. I was certain that Carlos heard it as well, because he suddenly started cheerleading again.

As the days passed, Oona's condition deteriorated. When she began to vomit, I suggested some investigations, then held my breath. Oona and Carlos both agreed. I exhaled.

It is never easy to give bad news, but there are times when it is even more difficult than usual. This was one of them. Oona was in renal failure, likely from tumor compression of her ureters, and had a partial bowel obstruction. Carlos's first words were, "What do we do to fix it? Don't worry Oona, this is just a little glitch, right doc?" Do you know that feeling you get as the roller coaster dives straight down towards the ground? That's what I felt. Oona looked at me. Her moist eyes revealed two messages. One was, "Tell me what I want to know," and the other was, "Don't lie to me."

As gently as I could, I explained, "Unfortunately, this is more than a little glitch." I spent a great deal of time describing what was likely going on medically. We could get an ultrasound done immediately. Oona and Carlos were comfortable with the plan. This surprised me initially, but I then realized upon further conversation that although they had heard the facts, they had interpreted them into a palatable situation. It unfortunately bore little resemblance to reality.

There was hydronephrosis on the ultrasound, and the couple did opt for nephrostomy tubes. It was one of those days when if something could go wrong, it did go wrong. Oona's procedure was delayed, and when they finally got to her, they had to try twice to insert the tube. This increased the pain associated with the procedure. To make matters worse, her creatinine did not decrease with the one tube, and she required a second.

I dreaded being the bearer of this news. I like to tell people how well something went and that all the pain was worth it, not that they need to endure more, without a guarantee of benefit in return. When I talked to Oona about the severity of her creatinine level, she looked so fragile.

I went home that night feeling not "right with the world." I realized that I was a lot like Oona, and that what was happening to her could happen to me. *Would I turn to a herbalist if I got cancer? Would I hear expert after expert say the same thing and not accept it?* I really didn't know what I would do.

The team on the palliative care unit viewed Oona as denying the severity of her situation and appeared to have a need to help her "face reality." I was uncomfortable with this. Some of the nurses were annoyed with me for not pushing a Do Not Resuscitate (DNR) order. I knew that if Oona required resuscitation, she would likely not survive, and while Oona knew this as well, she still wanted it. One of the nurses wrote in the chart that when she inquired of Oona if she wanted "everything done," that "Oona unfortunately replied yes." I find it so odd that we ask patients, "Do you want everything done?" and expect them to say no.

Ultimately, the team believed that Oona should not be on the unit since she was not in "a palliative mode" and was refusing to agree to a DNR order. The team sentiment was that Oona was dying, and that if she could not come to terms with that reality, then the bed should be available to someone who could.

Surprisingly, Oona valued the care she was receiving and the quiet atmosphere of the unit. She enjoyed the nurturing disposition of the nurses and felt that she belonged. I was unaware of this at the time, but Oona was the first to challenge the dogma of palliative care and was challenging me to be a lot more flexible. I found myself agreeing with her. She was a palliative patient and deserved our help despite her holding onto the hope of a miracle.

Three days after her second nephrostomy tube, she improved and requested another surgical opinion. They had heard that a surgeon located in a neighboring community was very skilled and aggressive and would attempt things others would not. This would be the fourth opinion. I was sure that the surgeon's response would be the same as the three previous opinions, that surgery was not possible. I was wrong.

I now had a patient on the palliative care unit that was not only a full code, but was also still getting treatment. The surgeon told Oona and Carlos that he felt that the tumor could be de-bulked, but not cured. All Carlos and Oona heard was that it could be "cut out." They were convinced that once the surgery got rid of the majority of the tumor, the herbal medication would be able to eradicate the remainder.

Oona was going home until the time of her surgery. She was radiant. When Oona was discharged, I felt positive about our rising rapport. I offered to have the palliative care outreach team visit her at home. In the flash of that moment, something changed. Oona looked at me bewildered and hurt. "I'm not palliative, I'm going to beat this." Oh no, the roller coaster again. I had the sense that nothing I would ever do or say would be good enough.

I visited Oona only once in the hospital, immediately after her debulking surgery.

"Hello," I smiled.

"Don't worry, she's only visiting," Carlos promised her. While Carlos' statement was accurate, none of us knew how our lives would intersect in the future.

Dori Seccareccia, Judith Belle Brown and Tanya Thornton

Postoperatively, Oona healed quickly, and from a surgical standpoint, the debulking operation was a success. I wondered how Oona's definition of success aligned with that of the surgeon. I never asked her. The gynecologic oncologists insisted that Oona involve the palliative care team again. She reluctantly agreed to call if the pain flared. A few months elapsed before the outreach team was asked to see Oona for recurring abdominal discomfort. It must have been fate, because I was on call for the community.

At their home, Carlos greeted me apprehensively, looking fatigued, but determined not to show it. "Oona has some tummy pain. We had Chinese food last night. I suspect it didn't agree with her, that's all," he commented as he led the way upstairs to the bedroom. Oona was lying down. Despite her elegant dressing gown and meticulous make-up, she looked uncomfortable. I prayed that I'd be able to help and that it was not what I feared – a progression of her disease. Clinically I felt that she had a partial bowel obstruction. Carlos disagreed: "Listen, doc, all she needs is some pain meds. No tests, no hospital, just medication. Can you do that?"

I explained, "It would be very helpful to have some blood work and X-rays to sort out what is causing the pain." Somehow Oona found the strength to forcefully shake her head no. She did have bowel sounds and had passed some stool, so we had time. I knew that it was not "good medicine" to give pain medication without a diagnosis, but I also felt that I was going to have to live with it. I implored Carlos to notify me immediately if Oona's condition deteriorated. The pain medication eased her furrowed brow. Oona was seeing the gynecologic oncologist in a few days. I remember worrying that he would think I was a "bad doctor" for treating the patient without the proper work-up. My "community consult" concluded, but my concerns about Oona did not recede.

A few months passed before our paths crossed again. This time, Oona had taken a turn for the worse. She had been experiencing back pain and leg weakness for a couple of weeks. Oona decided to only tell her herbalist, who informed her that he anticipated this outcome. Her symptoms, he explained, were a result of the compounds he had given her to break down the remaining cancer and now her body was washing it out of her system. So

Oona took these signs of spinal cord compression as a good thing and not as the ominous warning of impending disaster.

It was not until she became paralyzed that Carlos took her to the hospital. By then it was too late. Oona received emergency radiation therapy and when she did not respond, she received surgery for decompression. Oona was then transferred to the palliative care unit. Oona had agreed to the transfer, as she had regarded the unit in the past as "a safe and quiet environment to recuperate." She also believed it was a temporary measure. Oona was convinced she would walk again. And so was Carlos. I attempted to be honest without destroying hope.

After a few weeks of being on the unit, and not gaining any strength in her legs, I began to notice that Oona's words of determination were the same, but her voice had a growing echo of doubt. The stronger her doubt became, the more Carlos responded in his role of cheerleader. One Saturday, he took Oona on a day pass to the park to watch the rollerbladers. He intended to inspire her to walk and yes, eventually get on rollerblades. When Oona returned from that outing, she seemed to have aged 10 years in 10 hours.

Carlos was not ready to hear, let alone accept, Oona's change of heart. He felt that she was just tired and insisted that we promote a more positive attitude regarding the future and her ability to walk. As Oona became more lethargic and confused, Carlos insisted it was the result of the pain medication and that it be decreased. I was beside myself. Oona needed the pain medication. Her symptoms were due to progression of the disease, and not just the result of medications. Carlos did not want further tests for fear of what they might show. In contrast, Oona was starting to acknowledge that she would never walk again.

During her time on the palliative care unit, my role changed from being in charge of the inpatient unit to being solely focused on community consults. I was no longer primarily responsible for Oona's care. I told myself that it would not make a difference. I would still see her and be involved. It felt so awkward though. When I would think of something that might help, I couldn't just write an order. I was feeling out of control. During this time, Oona deteriorated. She finally agreed to some tests, which confirmed that the cancer had spread to her brain and liver.

Suddenly Carlos' attitude changed completely, and he only wanted Oona to be comfortable. As Oona became aware of this shift in Carlos, it caused her to become agitated. Sitting quietly with Oona one night, she began to share her mounting fears. "Carlos has given up hope," she said. "We believed together in the miracle – I was going to beat cancer. But now I am alone in this." Oona paused, then her voice changed. "He won't take me home, you know. He's cast me off!" She turned to face the window. I stole a glimpse at her reflection just as the tear she was trying to conceal slid over her gaunt cheekbone.

"He'll be upset for a while after I'm gone, but he'll carry on. He'll find someone to fill the void. I'll be replaced and life will go on." The dam holding back the tears finally gave way, and they streamed down. Without reservation, she sobbed until her frail frame was spent. Throughout all this, I sat silent, holding her hand. She looked up and admitted, "It's driving me crazy to think these thoughts, but when I'm alone in here I can't help it – my mind imagines a future without me in it."

Two days before dying, Oona insisted on going to physiotherapy. She was sleeping 20 hours a day now, and her well-seen skeleton wore only pale and dry skin. It was as though all the muscle and fat had evaporated. Yet she endured being positioned onto the exercise bicycle, and pedaled slowly for less than a minute. The staff fought back tears. Part of me felt ripped apart watching this, and part of me understood completely. Yes, death was inevitable, but she didn't have to like it or get used to it. Why should she? She had suffered many hardships and had always transformed disadvantage into advantage. She had never hurt anyone and had worked hard to raise her family and be a good teacher and take care of herself. She respected and loved life, and her actions lived up to her beliefs. So why should she lay down peacefully and accept this? For whose benefit would it be? More likely it would be for the people who were uncomfortable watching her struggle. But Oona had to die for Oona, and not for others.

Oona, you taught me so much. You taught me not to be afraid to fight for what you believe in, even when others disagree. Not to bow down to certainty, because no one can predict the future. You had a year of life that you would not have had if you would have listened to the majority and not had the surgery. You taught me not to define for others what is or is not palliative care, but to listen, both actively and compassionately. You taught me not to be afraid to accompany someone on their journey with suffering and never to be bold enough to think that I know what is best for someone else.

I went to Oona's memorial service. I don't go to many, but I do go to some. They are chosen selfishly, for my sense of closure and for my own peace. People always ask me how I can possibly do what I do. I smile to myself and think that I have the best job in the world. I am in a sacred and privileged position to learn about life from people who have had to do a lot more living and struggling than I. They give so much more to me than I can ever give to them. I hope that I have the strength to use this knowledge wisely and to share it whenever I can.

27 Growing Into A Mom

Lisa Graves, Judith Belle Brown and Tanya Thornton

"Absolutely *not!* Never!" Aimee retorted. Her black curls bounced with angry energy as she whipped her head from side to side. "I told you mom, doctors are all the same, let's go."

"It's okay if you choose not to have the RhoGAM today, we can discuss it next time," Dr. Saang replied, trying to regain composure and salvage what she could of the first prenatal visit.

"Not ever. No RhoGAM. Don't you get it – taking RhoGAM would be more traumatic than what I've already gone through," Aimee reiterated adamantly. "It goes against my beliefs and values. How could I face my family, my sisters, my friends, my church? You just don't understand."

"You're right, I don't really understand, but I'll try to. Let's start over." Dr. Saang sighed as she sat down into her office chair and swiveled to face Aimee. "Okay, since this is our first visit together, tell me about yourself."

Dr. Saang settled in for what she thought would be a long, drawn-out description of Aimee's life, and was immediately surprised to discover how articulate and insightful Aimee was, despite her youth of 18 years. She resembled her older sister, Clara, who was also a patient of Dr. Saang's. They shared the same high cheekbones and broad facial features, but Aimee's dark eyes, although shining with determination, were often downcast during their discussion.

Dr. Saang learned that Aimee's pregnancy was the result of a rape. On the advice of her mother, Aimee consulted a physician early on in her pregnancy. To her horror, he encouraged her to terminate the pregnancy, insisting that she was too young and the circumstances were too difficult. She fled from the office and never returned. As part of a close-knit Jehovah's Witness community, her sisters and friends had provided support and advice along the way. But now she needed medical expertise to prepare her for the delivery. She gave in to Clara's pleas to at least talk with her family physician. Her sister trusted Dr. Saang and finally, Aimee agreed to a visit. As that day approached, Aimee became terrified that this new physician, like the first, would not respect her faith. She understood fully that by not receiving RhoGAM to prevent isoimmunization, she might never have another child. She accepted this without reservation. What she couldn't accept was a blood product.

Throughout their conversation, Aimee looked down at the office carpet. She fought hard to restrain the sob welling in her throat. "I didn't want to be a mom, you know. Not now, maybe not ever. But now I have no choice. I don't want this baby, I don't know if I'll ever be able to love it." The sob broke, her chest heaved.

"Now Aimee, we've discussed this," her mom interjected, "you know I'll take care of the baby for you." Her mom looked pointedly at Dr. Saang and said, "The family will love it, even if Aimee cannot."

Observing the interaction between mother and daughter, Dr. Saang realized that although Aimee was a young adult, she was suffocating from the care doled out by the older family members. She was surrounded by strong and independent women. Although it was this care that had supported her thus far, it was clear that if Aimee were to embark on this new journey of motherhood, she would need to become more autonomous. Defining Aimee as an adult needed to occur early so that her mother would understand her own role. "I'd like to chat with Aimee alone now, and do a brief physical. Is that okay, Aimee?"

"Yes, that's fine," Aimee nodded.

"Okay, I'll be in the waiting room if you need me, honey." Her mother leaned in, gave her a gentle kiss on her crown and quietly left the exam room.

"Aimee, you're 18, you're an adult, but I understand, this is not how you envisioned your young adulthood. However, because you are an adult, *you* run the show here. As your doctor, I am going to listen to you, not to your mother. Do you understand that?" Aimee nodded again. "It's wonderful you have such a supportive family, and most pregnant first-time moms want advice from their own mom – so it's appropriate and realistic for her to be involved, but *you* can decide how much your mom is to be involved. Okay?"

"Thanks," Aimee said, smiling.

"On that note, I'm here to support you too. Women who have been sexually assaulted find healing when they talk it through with a counselor. Have you had the opportunity to do that Aimee?"

"I'm fine, I don't need a counselor."

"If you haven't met with someone yet, it might be a good time to chat, before the baby comes, while you still have time to yourself."

"Counselors wouldn't understand."

"Who would understand?"

Aimee sat silent, shrugged her shoulders, then whispered, "Maybe an elder at the church."

"That's likely true. I could see how they would understand the decisions you've made. Are you sure they'd have the experience and expertise to help you deal with the rape?"

"I don't want to talk about that. Dealing with the baby is hard enough. You say you're here to support me and you want me to trust you – then let it go. Trust me when I tell you I'll talk about it when I'm ready."

Dr. Saang sat quiet for a few moments. She realized that in order to demonstrate that she respected Aimee, with all of her reservations and fears for her, she would have to agree to let it go.

"Okay, should we listen to the baby's heartbeat now then?"

Aimee broke into a big smile and replied, "Yeah, that'd be awesome. Thanks."

As Dr. Saang squeezed the jelly onto Aimee's protruding belly, her thoughts wandered. She wondered why Aimee was resistant to discuss the context of the rape. Clara had told Dr. Saang in confidence that Aimee's description of the assault was vague enough to suggest that the assailant may have been an acquaintance. Her sister had already warned Dr. Saang that Aimee opposed any attempt to delve further into the events. She had not sought prenatal care in fear that she would be forced to deal with the trauma she was not ready to acknowledge. Furthermore, Aimee did not wish to pursue legal action against the assailant, giving rise to the query that the intercourse was consensual. Given the incongruence with Aimee's religious beliefs, the safest psychological posture was to maintain the guise of a sexual assault rather than face the disapproval by her family and her faith. Dr. Saang was cognizant of an aura of conspiracy, but confronting Aimee about the discrepancies in her story would have shattered the support she so clearly needed.

"There it is – the fast one – that's your baby's heartbeat," Dr. Saang said, smiling down at Aimee. "It's a healthy one, and a busy one, moving all over the place here."

As Dr. Saang turned off the doptone and helped Aimee sit up, she reminded Aimee, "You're insightful enough to understand the limitations and challenges of seeking counseling within your community. However, if that's what you prefer, I think it is better that you talk to them, rather than keep it bottled up. It will help you be a better mom, and help you heal." Dr. Saang put a hand on Aimee's arm. "And if you ever change your mind and want someone else to talk to, well you know I am here for you."

"I'm glad I came today." Aimee admitted, sliding down off the exam table. "When should I come back for my next checkup?"

"I'll see you in two weeks," Dr. Saang replied, handing her an appointment card.

In the end, it appeared that living with the shame of the sexual assault was easier to bear than the silent disgrace Aimee feared would haunt her soul if she had chosen to hide the pregnancy by aborting. The refusal to accept RhoGAM may well have meant that this baby was the only child she would have. At 18 years of age, it was hard to believe that Aimee was capable of understanding the ramifications of this decision. Yet Aimee repeatedly asserted her position that her beliefs were more important to her than the issues surrounding her future reproductive health.

As Aimee's physician, Dr. Saang came to terms with her patient's decisions and accepted them as part of whom Aimee was, informed by a knowledge and understanding of her patient's context and values. For Aimee, she realized that the duty of the physician was to counsel and inform, but that the final decisions would always be hers. Furthermore, her decision to seek counsel from within her community, when she was ready, was acknowledged.

In a similar vein, Aimee and her mom reached a common understanding of their roles in Aimee's prenatal care. Aimee's mom, although relishing the caretaker position, acquiesced to Dr. Saang's counsel, which emphasized the need for Aimee to become responsible for her own health and well-being. Although she continued to accompany Aimee on prenatal appointments, she did agree to let Aimee have the privacy needed to discuss issues with her physician, and only came into the exam room when invited by Aimee.

In order to forge ahead as a young adult and new mom, Dr. Saang recognized the need for Aimee to act and decide independently. Through the process of finding common ground, Dr. Saang, her mom and Aimee each matured. Dr. Saang learned to accept a patient's decisions, even if they were contrary to her own principles and understanding. Aimee's mom became cognizant of the value in relinquishing control in lieu of a supportive presence. Finally, Aimee grew into the label "mom" – in more ways than one.

28 "You're Not Listening to Me!"

Jill Konkin and Judith Belle Brown

The first patient of the morning was a young woman, Reta Grath, who had been seen the previous night in the emergency room. This was expected, as Dr. Bishop had asked Reta to call the clinic as soon as it opened to secure one of the appointment times allocated for urgent cases. When Dr. Bishop entered the room, sat down and asked Reta how she was feeling, Reta immediately blurted out, "I'm very angry. I don't think you've been listening to me." Dr. Bishop was stunned.

The night before, 30-year-old Reta presented to the emergency department with a history of left-sided chest pain that had persisted for almost a month. It was sharp and occasionally took her breath away. "Most importantly," Reta explained, "the pain is interfering with my sleep. I have trouble falling asleep and once I finally get to sleep the pain will wake me up." She was not short of breath, had no cough or fever, and the pain did not radiate. But Reta looked exhausted, her face pale and sunken. Her frustration was apparent as she said, "The pain never really goes away."

Dr. Bishop knew that about a year ago Reta had discovered a lump in her left breast during the third trimester of her pregnancy. She had been sent for investigation and an ultrasound and needle biopsy were conducted. The lump was observed to be a fibroadenoma, and Reta was booked for a mammogram and repeat ultrasound about five months after the birth of her daughter. However, Reta had cancelled her appointment at the Breast Center, located almost 250 miles away, and she had not rebooked.

Reta indicated that her lump had not changed in size or consistency. On examination, there was a 1 cm by 1.5 cm, mobile, smooth, slightly tender mass in the upper outer quadrant of the left breast. There was chest wall tenderness over ribs two and three at the anterior axillary line. The lungs were clear. There was nothing else to find on examination.

"Reta, are you concerned that the pain is related to the breast lump?" inquired Dr. Bishop. Reta quickly responded, "No, not all." Indeed Reta was unable to articulate any fears about what the pain might be. "I'm just very tired. I'm not getting any sleep because of the constant pain," she reiterated. Her voice revealed her sense of growing desperation. "It's a real struggle to get up in the morning. But I have no choice. I have to get ready for work, plus get Tamara fed, dressed and off to day care. That's a real struggle, 'cause that little lass has a mind of her own!" Reta suddenly paused, wincing in pain. "See," she said, catching her breath, "it comes on just like that!"

"Well, Reta," Dr. Bishop began and was abruptly interrupted by the wail of incoming ambulances transporting casualties from a five-car pile-up on the freeway. Both their heads shifted in the direction of the ambulance bay. Dr. Bishop tightened as she imagined the trauma she might face in the coming hours; Reta anxiously turned back to her physician seeking relief. Rapidly assessing the situation, Dr. Bishop decided to order a non-narcotic analgesic and a heat pack for Reta. "Listen, Reta," she explained speedily, "we'll try this and see how you feel in the next half an hour or so to see if you feel any better. If you don't, then we will try something else. Okay?" Dr. Bishop promptly left Reta alone on the stretcher, in pain.

Although the blare of the ambulance sirens was now silent, the noise and chaos of the emergency room intensified as the accident victims were being triaged and treated. It took much longer than a half hour before Dr. Bishop was able to return to Reta's bedside. "Are you feeling any better?" Dr. Bishop asked and then added, "Sorry it took so long to get back to you, pretty crazy here tonight." Dr. Bishop smiled slightly. "Anyway, how do you feel now?"

"I'm okay," responded Reta in a quiet, almost inaudible voice. "I have to get home," she stated anxiously, "Tamara's been at the neighbor's for hours." Reta's tone suddenly changed as she said, "I must get her home into her own crib where she feels safe," she concluded in a strident manner.

"Okay Reta, but here is another dose of analgesic to take home with you in case you needed something more during the night, and please call first thing in the morning to come in for follow-up," Dr. Bishop responded as Reta swung her legs off the stretcher and rapidly gathered her belongings.

Now as they sat together the following day, Dr. Bishop experienced Reta's expression of anger towards her as unwarranted. Dr. Bishop considered herself to be a caring and compassionate physician who was patient-centered. An emotional smorgasbord passed through her mind – anger, confusion and disappointment in herself, to name a few. Last night's encounter may not have been optimal, but Reta's response was unexpected.

When anger and defensiveness become omnipresent in the patient-doctor relationship, it can render finding common ground an impossible task. Dr. Bishop took in a silent deep breath and asked Reta to continue. As Reta unloaded her anger, a series of issues emerged that shed light on the mismatch in expectations and how a failure to find common ground had occurred during the last few encounters.

Reta's initial feeling of being rebuffed by Dr. Bishop emanated from a visit during a well-baby check for her daughter a month ago. As the visit was winding up, Reta asked, "I need to come in for a complete examination soon. When would that be?"

"Well, the waiting list for complete examinations is three months long," Dr. Bishop explained, but before she could continue with her usual qualifier of the availability of an earlier appointment for a specific problem, Tamara let out a sharp cry. She had caught her finger between a chair and the desk. Tamara's sobs filled the room, and both Dr. Bishop's and Reta's attention was sufficiently distracted such that the invitation to come in sooner was never extended. Reta felt unheard and rejected.

As Reta catalogued the mounting concerns that had fuelled her current anger, the story unfolded. During Reta's explanation, it became evident that a significant amount of her anger was related to her ambivalence and ultimate fear of narcotic analgesics. "You may not know this, but I had a serious cocaine habit that I have struggled to overcome," she explained in a hostile tone. Her physical posture revealed her sense of shame and humiliation. Reta was very worried that she might become addicted to narcotics if she used them for pain control. At the same time, Reta was convinced that perhaps only narcotics could control her pain until its source could be located and addressed. She confirmed that she did not think that the pain came from the breast lump, though on further questioning she did admit that she was more concerned about the lump than she had been willing to admit.

Reta agreed to make an appointment with the Breast Center to further investigate her breast lump as well as to have some other investigations done. She was also given a prescription for a small amount of a narcotic analgesic. The proper use of analgesics was discussed, and Reta assured herself that she would only use the narcotic for pain. She agreed to come back in one week to report on her pain and to review the results of the investigations. Dr. Bishop thanked her for her honesty in expressing her anger and for her willingness to work things out.

A week later, Reta reported that she was now sleeping much better and the responsibilities of caring for Tamara felt less arduous. She had been surprised at how little analgesic she had needed and was less anxious about becoming addicted. "You know," Reta volunteered, "it was real hard for me to find the courage to confront you at our last visit but I had to!" Reta, looking reflective stated, "It made no sense for me to simply go off and choke back my anger." Then, shifting gears, Reta proudly announced, "I have an appointment at the Breast Center. I have a ride arranged to the Center and I got day care all set for Tamara, so I don't have to get all fussed and worried about her!" Reta's sense of accomplishment in achieving these tasks and fulfilling her role in setting the process of her care in motion was monumental.

At their next visit a month later, Reta was in good spirits. The Breast Center appointment had gone well. The breast lump was benign. Reta was comfortable with the diagnosis and did not want to have it excised at this time. Her anxiety had been put to rest and so too had Dr. Bishop's.

At the end of the visit, Reta gave Dr. Bishop a hug. "Thanks Dr. B. for being willing to listen to me even when I was angry and not just shrugging me off," said Reta with a bright and shining smile. "And," her eyelashes fluttered and her voice slightly cracked as she concluded, "thanks for being willing to take the time to help me figure out what gets me so riled!"

This story of a patient and her doctor illustrates the enduring relevance of the patient-physician relationship in the pivotal process of finding common ground. Reta found the courage to express her anger because she had known Dr. Bishop to not only be a caring physician but also a doctor who would invite her to mutually engage in identifying her problems or concerns. Furthermore, past experience had shown Reta how Dr. Bishop had, for the most part, encouraged her to be an active participant in decisions about her care. Thus the history of their past successes at finding common ground prevented the process from unraveling during this challenging time.

29 A Sad Refrain

Jana Malhotra and Judith Belle Brown

Eileen was my patient, and these were her first words to me. "I am in pain, so much pain. You have no idea what my life has been like. I am 82 years old." I had just recently taken over her care at the local nursing home in our small, rural community. I didn't know very much about her when I met her for the initial time, only what her chart revealed: past medical history, list of medications, allergies, next of kin. From this list, I knew that she was on an extraordinary amount of pain medication that had slowly escalated over the years.

My other source of information was amply supplied by the nursing home staff. The nurses, clearly exasperated, implored me: "Please do something about her!", "We can't handle it!", "We're burned out!", "We just can't deal with her anymore!" When I popped into the dining area of the nursing home to grab a quick coffee before starting rounds, I was assailed by a torrent of comments by the dietary staff. "She says our food is causing her pain!" was the collective refrain. Armed with these comments and her short medical history, I went to meet Eileen.

She was demanding, she did have a lot of complaints and she did create a difficult atmosphere for the staff at the nursing home. However, Eileen suffered. She had chronic pain from her osteoarthritis, which she felt was only alleviated with high-dose narcotic medication. She worried about her family and their health, which were not inconsequential concerns given the hereditary cardiomyopathy that affected the family.

On our first visit, Eileen shared some of her past. "My daughter has cardiomyophy, you know. It's a terrible, terrible disease. We're not sure where it came from – the doctors think maybe from her father. He died young – was only fifty-three years old. That was a while ago, back in the seventies. I guess they didn't really know much about it back then. When he died, they didn't tell me why, I don't think they knew. And then my son got it. He died at twenty-seven. I looked after him while he was sick. Looked after my husband, then my son. They both died."

Eileen's family history revealed the source of her loss and sorrow. Fighting back her grief, she had committed herself to caring for her family. "I did everything for them, for my family. I looked after all of them myself, on my own," she said with a tone of pride in her voice. "I had to work part-time at the hardware store to make ends meet, but I did it. I have worked hard all of my life." Eileen paused, a look of hurt transforming her face, "I don't think they really understand that here. They just think I'm a crabby old woman."

It was not easy being Eileen's physician over the months that passed. Her expectations were not always realistic, she could be manipulative with me and the other staff, and she refused specialist care because of the fear that they would try to decrease her narcotic medications. There were days when she was my "heartsink" patient – days when I didn't really think I could handle the required interaction with her one more time.

As soon as I walked through the door of the nursing home, Eileen would quickly make her way up to the nursing station and say, "Doctor, I don't want to be a bother, but I need to talk to you ..." and she would stand and wait for me.

At each encounter, Eileen showered me with complaints of her pain. "I am in pain all of the time. From the moment that I wake up, until I go to sleep, and even then, I'm up all night with the pain," she would moan. Then Eileen would adamantly state, "I never took painkillers before. I started when I got here. When was that? Oh, it's been a long time, ever since my last surgery. They won't do another one, have I told you that? On account of all my problems. I went to see the surgeon, and he said that there is nothing he can do. My hip is all degenerative or whatever they call it." Eileen would pause for a moment, and her eyes wide with anticipation, she would ask, "Does that have something to do with my nerves? I think it does." As quickly, she would return to the litany of her pain complaints "I can feel the pain in the nerves. It starts here, in my back, and travels down my leg, past my knee. Sharp, shooting pain. You wouldn't believe it. I'm not one to complain, but this pain is bad. I suffer so much."

My frustration stemmed partly from my own inability to meet Eileen's demands. I would never be able to bring her pain level down to her required "zero out of ten." I would never cure her chronic cough, her difficulty sleeping, or her itchy legs, as she expected me to. There had been several failed attempts to discuss my definition of "reasonable" care expectations for Eileen. However, she clung to her "Doctor, please help me" refrain. Didn't I go to medical school to help the patient that needs my assistance?

Several months after I had been caring for Eileen, she told me about a recent chapter in the family's legacy of cardiomyopathy. This time, it was her 23-year-old granddaughter. "I have a lot on my mind." Eileen's eyes filled with tears. She paused momentarily to regain her composure. "Did I tell you about my granddaughter? She was just diagnosed with the cardiomyopathy too – last week." Eileen began to choke up again. "She's my other son's daughter. We thought she had got away without it since her dad is okay. I don't know what happened. I guess she got it from my husband. She's so young." Eileen was now sobbing uncontrollably and began her woeful refrain. "Dear, I'm in so much pain, I know you will help me. You will help me, won't you?"

It was abundantly clear to me how her physical and emotional pain were inextricably linked: a lifetime of sorrow and loss. The recent news of her granddaughter was devastating. But as she had in the past, Eileen translated her psyche pain into physical pain. I doubted I could reverse this pattern, so I set out to find other means to address Eileen's pain.

I decided to establish a routine with Eileen – predictable and constant. I saw her every week, at the beginning of my rounds. I met her in her room, she told me about her pain, her shoulder, her back, her nerves, her daughter and granddaughter. I listened to her sad refrain time and time again, "I try not to be a bother, but I have pain. No one seems to understand. Except for you, doctor. I know you will help me. Will you help me?" Each time I would tell her that she was doing a wonderful job handling all of her burdens. I agreed that she has a lot of pain, more than any one person should have. Sometimes I have looked at a new spot that hurt on her toe, and sometimes I have prescribed a hot water bottle for the pain. I listened to her concerns and tried to ease her sorrow.

So we work together, balancing on this tightrope. I'm not sure if we will fall off at some point, but for now, I'm grateful that we have achieved this fine balance.

30 Unexplored Territory – Part 1

Joshua Shadd and Judith Belle Brown

Marcus was almost a typical 19 year old – scrawny, baggy clothes, unkempt hair and restless eyes. He and his girlfriend, Angie, had recently moved to town in order to attend the local community college – he for a career in IT, she as an esthetician. Marcus enjoyed school and loved Angie, but his real passion was playing his bass guitar. "That's how I decompress," he explained. He was like his freshmen classmates in almost every way – except that Marcus had undergone more cancer treatments than anyone Dr. Boice had ever met.

Marcus's previous family physician introduced him to Dr. Boice via a referral letter. Marcus was diagnosed with Wilms' tumor of the left kidney at age six. Despite aggressive, curative-intent therapy, his first recurrence appeared at age 12. Since then, Marcus had undergone seven more operations in addition to multiple cycles of chemo and radiation therapy. The letter identified pain as Marcus's primary concern and cautioned that much effort had been expended to find an acceptable analgesic regimen. The unspoken message was clear: common ground had not been found easily. Medication changes were risky.

The notes from the local pediatric oncologist added valuable insights. Marcus declined a repeat chest X-ray to assess progression of his known lung metastases. When the oncologist raised questions about the future, Marcus closed the discussion. Further chemotherapy, it seemed, was not in his plans.

Dr. Boice's goal going into his first encounter with Marcus was simple: to build rapport. It was clear that Marcus's malignancy, while not causing major problems at the moment, was progressing. Marcus was new in town with no support except his girlfriend, and there were storm clouds on the horizon. Dr. Boice suspected their relationship would be an important one for Marcus in the not-too-distant future.

Marcus attended his first appointment, like all of his appointments, alone. He discussed his story comfortably, often recalling specific names and dates. He was obviously well-practiced in providing his medical history. When asked about his family, Marcus confirmed what Dr. Boice had read in his chart: parents separated but supportive, one healthy younger sister. Marcus didn't elaborate further. When asked how he felt about his illness, Marcus politely but unequivocally declined to discuss it.

Marcus's analgesic regimen was the kind that raises a yellow flag – regular use of short-acting oxycodone alongside scheduled long-acting oxycodone.

During that first visit, Marcus reinforced the message from the referral letter – it had been very difficult to find an adequate analgesic strategy, and he wasn't interested in changing anything. He was greatly relieved when Dr. Boice confirmed his willingness to continue prescribing his current pain medications.

Marcus came to clinic once per month. He was always alone. The visits quickly fell into a pattern. He would talk about what he was learning in his networking or web design course. He mentioned his girlfriend often, but his family never. They would discuss his pain. At every other visit, Dr. Boice would gently probe about Marcus's emotional state and coping. Marcus would immediately close the door, and Dr. Boice would respect this by not bringing it up at the next visit. As Marcus was functioning well overall, this defense mechanism seemed to be adaptive and Dr. Boice saw no reason to challenge it. Marcus ended every visit the same way: "Thanks for being there for me, oc."

When Dr. Boice proposed initiating an adjuvant analgesic for the neuropathic component of his pain, Marcus had only one question: "Will I still be able to play my bass?" Marcus's fluctuating degree of engagement with his music proved to be Dr. Boice's one narrow window into Marcus's illness experience. The pain improved somewhat, and his opioid dose remained stable. At the beginning of the winter term, things seemed to be going well. Marcus decided to pick up an elective course in biology, and at each clinic visit he wanted to learn a new medical term to take back to his professor.

It was late January when the clinic nurse interrupted Dr. Boice between appointments. "Marcus called," she began with a concerned expression. "He says that he needs another prescription because he dropped his pills in the toilet." Dr. Boice's heart sank. Marcus might as well have said "the dog ate my homework." This could make it much more difficult to help Marcus. Dr. Boice asked him to come to clinic that afternoon.

During that visit, Dr. Boice expressed his concerns. "Marcus, I've been your doctor for almost six months now, and you've never given me reason to doubt you. But I need to tell you how concerned I am about the loss of these pills."

Marcus was visibly upset. "Doc, I'm not lying to you! You have to trust me on this – you have to! I'm not selling my pills! Look, I brought in the pills that fell into the toilet. I can use them if I need to."

Dr. Boice's response was gentle but firm. "Marcus, I do trust you and I will give you a prescription today, but you need to understand that I won't be able to do so again."

"Thanks, doc." Marcus sighed. "You gotta believe me. I wouldn't lie to you."

Marcus seemed relieved as he left the office. Despite his statement of reassurance to Marcus, something still didn't seem right to Dr. Boice. Marcus had given over the pills recovered from the toilet, but they were far fewer than needed to get to his next scheduled prescription. Dr. Boice asked the clinic nurse to call the pharmacy to confirm what had been dispensed. This time, she hung up the phone with a smile. It turned out the pharmacy had dispensed only a two-week instead of his usual four-week supply. Marcus's story was vindicated. Dr. Boice was relieved. Trust in their relationship was important for him too.

COMPONENT IV

Enhancing the Patient-Doctor Relationship

Moira Stewart and Judith Belle Brown

Lord Byron wrote: "Sorrows are our best education. A person can see further through a tear than a telescope." For the clinician bearing witness to suffering, the patient-doctor relationship can provide the best education; the doctor can see more through a tear than a stethoscope.

The patient-doctor relationship is the bedrock of the patient-centered clinical method. In this section, we examine some well-known conceptualizations of helping relationships including: compassion characterized by the attributes of empathy and caring; power; constancy; healing; self-awareness; and transference and countertransference.

COMPASSION, EMPATHY AND CARING

Empathy is a complex and important characteristic of the therapeutic relationship. In order to have compassion, empathy is a key ingredient – the capacity "to walk in another's shoes." Caring implies that the doctor is fully present and engaged with the patient. The doctor and patient are interconnected in such a deep way that the doctor can fully immerse him- or herself in the concerns of the patient (Montgomery 1993). Intense caring moments in relationships involve mutual recognition on the part of patient and practitioner and a reciprocal learning of both individuals (Frank 1991; Watson 1985; Suchman and Matthews 1988). Boundaries may be much more blurred than in the traditional, distanced, one-way relationship. However, the closeness restores patients' sense of connectedness to the human race, a connectedness that may have been broken by their physical, emotional or spiritual suffering (Belenky *et al.* 1986; Candib 1988; Cassell 1991; Vaillant 2008).

Compassion, empathy and caring are paramount in the clinician's work with vulnerable populations (Redelmeier *et al.* 2005; McWilliam *et al.* 1997; Pottie *et al.* 2005; Woolhouse *et al.* 2011). Calling forth these attributes may be a challenge when the patient's circumstances are horrific and are experienced as difficult for the physician to bear witness. Yet it is these very attributes that facilitate the doctor to serve a healing role.

POWER IN THE PATIENT-DOCTOR RELATIONSHIP

Power and control in the patient-doctor relationship have been examined in the literature for over 40 years. There is no doubt that the relationship that is the foundation for patient-centered care, as compared to the traditional relationship, demands a sharing of power and control between the doctor and the patient (Brody 1992). Other authors who have proposed models of patient-doctor relationships have variously described the state of high-patient control of decision-making as: mutuality (Szasz and Hollender 1956); the contractual relationship (Veatch 1972); the consumerist approach (Haug and Lavin 1983; Stewart and Roter 1989; Roter and Hall 1992). These approaches are similar but not identical to Component III – Finding Common Ground, as described previously. The quality of a relationship within which finding common ground is possible includes a readiness of doctor and patient to become partners in care. Their encounters are truly meetings between experts (Tuckett *et al.* 1985). The doctor is the medical expert; whereas the patient is the expert regarding his or her unique illness experience and life circumstances. In addition, each partnership is unique and may include permutations and combinations employing varying degrees of control along many dimensions and change over time. The balance of power may be altered based on the patient's particular needs and expectations.

CONTINUITY AND CONSTANCY

Continuity of care is longitudinal care delivered over time within the context of a long-term relationship between patient and physician. Loxtercamp has eloquently described the power of continuing relationships in this way: "Doctors who remain deeply connected to their patients will know the privilege, as will those who retain the capacity to listen, touch, tether ourselves to the wounds of others. In modest ways, we accomplish the utterly profound long before the prescription is filled or the blood test is taken. We profit by the patients' periodic return and by the mutual exchange of friendship, intimacy and trust" (Loxtercamp 2001, p 247).

System barriers and gaps in service within the health care system have resulted in serious disruptions in continuity of care. In addition, physicians burdened by increasing service demands and patient care responsibilities may consciously or unconsciously close doors, or – at worst – abandon patients. As the concept of continuity comes under threat, it remains the doctor's responsibility to be constant in his or her commitment to the well-being of the patient. Constancy as described by Cassell (1991) requires the clinician to provide "constant attention and [a] maintained presence" which brings "… that promised stability in the uncertain world of sickness arising from their relationship" (p. 78).

HEALING

The attributes of the doctor and the characteristics of the relationship are what make the patient-doctor relationship therapeutic. Like many other helping professionals, doctors perform an important role as healers, but healing the body and healing the person are not identical and often not simultaneous. The healing of a patient involves a process of restoring the patient's lost sense of connectedness, indestructibility and control. The healing process is "no more than allowing, causing or bringing to bear those things or forces for getting better that already exist in the patient" (Cassell 1991, p. 234).

For the most part, physicians see themselves as curers of patients' physical ills. They are less conscious of the need to restore patients to wellness by embracing the mandate to care and to heal. To heal is to restore a sense of coherence and wholeness after the disruption in a person's life that is caused by a serious illness. The physical disease may not be curable, but a healer can assist patients in regaining their emotional and spiritual equilibrium.

SELF-AWARENESS

In order to be compassionate, share power, remain a constant presence and ultimately to be a healer requires self-awareness on the part of the clinician. The use of self, and attending to the impact on self, both require a depth of self-knowledge. Personal insight is integral to the clinician's use of self in the patient-doctor relationship. Novack *et al.* (1997, p. 502) state: "Because physicians use themselves as instruments of diagnosis and therapy, personal awareness can help them to 'calibrate their instruments,' using themselves more effectively in these capacities."

Self-awareness can be a natural outgrowth of reflection on experience and sharing these reflections with colleagues, friends and family. It can be further enhanced by supervision or consultation, professional and personal development. Epstein *et al.* (1993) propose three possible venues for developing self-awareness: Balint groups, which were conceived by Michael and Enid Balint (Balint 1957); family of origin groups, stemming from the work of Murray Bowen (1976, 1978), which examine how individuals' families of origin influence their relationships with patients; and personal awareness groups, which have evolved from the contributions of Carl Rogers (1961). Other authors endorse the important knowledge and understanding imparted in insights offered by the writing of narratives (Borkan *et al.* 1999; Greenhalgh and Hurwitz 1998; Brown *et al.* 2002; Ofri 2005; Groopman 2008; Nuland 2010; Cameron 2011; Charon 2004, 2006, 2007; Frank 1995, 2004).

The development of self-awareness requires clinicians to know their strengths and weaknesses. Self-awareness and self-knowledge also have a positive value in that they promote and nurture the qualities of empathy, sensitivity, honesty, humility, compassion and caring in the physician. Self-knowledge is a lifelong journey, a process that is never complete. Epstein's (1999) conceptualization of "mindful practice" raises the concept of physician self-awareness to a new level that is more complex and multi-faceted. He states: "This process of critical self-reflection depends on the presence of mindfulness. A mindful practitioner attends, in a nonjudgmental way, to his or her own physical and mental processes during ordinary everyday tasks to act with clarity and insight" (p. 833).

TRANSFERENCE AND COUNTERTRANSFERENCE

All human relationships, and in particular, therapeutic relationships, are influenced by the phenomena of transference and countertransference. Thus any discussion of the patient-doctor relationship that excluded these important psychological processes would be remiss. We do not intend to provide the reader with a detailed examination of transference and countertransference, instead what follows is a brief description. We feel that this is essential in order to define the parameters in which many of the dimensions, e.g. compassion, power, constancy, healing and self-awareness, of the patient-doctor relationship frequently occur.

Transference is a process whereby the patient unconsciously projects – onto individuals in his or her current life – thoughts, behaviors and emotional reactions that originate with other significant relationships from childhood onwards (Dubovsky 1981; Woods and Hollis 1990; Goldberg

2000). This can include feelings of love, hate, ambivalence and dependency. The greater the current attachment, such as a significant patient-doctor relationship, the more likely that transference will occur. Knowledge of the patient's transference reaction, either positive or negative, assists the doctor in understanding how the patient experiences his or her world and how past relationships influence current behavior. Also understanding the patient's transference reactions enhances the doctor's capacity for caring and can provide an emotionally corrective experience.

Countertransference, like transference, is an unconscious process that occurs when the doctor responds to patients in a manner similar to significant past relationships (Dubovsky 1981; Woods and Hollis 1990; Goldberg 2000). The origins and significance of doctors' countertransference are as varied and complex as their patients. We all struggle with unresolved issues from our past. Doctors need to be alert to what triggers certain reactions, e.g. unresolved personal issues, stress or value conflicts. It is here that self-awareness, coupled with the ability for self-observation during the consultation, is paramount.

The primary tool for effectively using transference and countertransference to aid and deepen the patient-physician relationship is physician self-awareness. Such self-knowledge is a requirement for the doctor's accurate recognition of both transference and countertransference. Self-evaluation and working with others may help doctors gain valuable insights that will ultimately strengthen relationships with patients and also increase their own comfort and satisfaction with the practice of medicine (Goldberg 2000).

CONCLUSION

The interactive components of the patient-centered clinical method occur within the ongoing relationship. The relationship is accomplished through a sustained partnership with a patient that includes compassion, sharing power, constancy and healing. Self-awareness promotes the clinician's deliberate and subjective use of transference and countertransference in the healing process.

Preview of the Narratives

As noted above, the patient-clinician relationship is the foundation of the patient-centered clinical method. The following narratives touch upon many qualities of this relationship – self-awareness, constancy, healing, transference and countertransference.

The first narrative in this section on the patient-doctor relationship is **Chapter 31**, the second half of Marcus's story. In this narrative, the patient-doctor relationship, the bedrock of patient-centered care, is put to a test. The final outcome is positive for both the patient and his doctor. But perhaps it is the physician, who through self-awareness learns the most – about himself.

Chapter 32 illustrates the invaluable role family physicians play at the end of life by providing advocacy and constancy. The family physician's active presence, amidst little hope, can be healing. It can restore losses and make one whole again.

The next five stories, **Chapter 33**, **Chapter 34**, **Chapter 35**, **Chapter 36** and **Chapter 37**, examine the patient-clinician relationship from the perspective of the physician. The first narrative explores how countertransference can be subtle, yet at the same time be very powerful and subsequently enhance the quality of the patient-doctor relationship. The next story reveals how the patient-doctor relationship can serve as a healing function for the physician as well as the patient. The third narrative, illustrating the component of the patient-doctor relationship, highlights how understanding the complex and dynamic interchange of transference and countertransference can be an important guide in the care of our patients. In this scenario it is a man who has suffered years of domestic abuse. What aids the clinician in her ability to therapeutically utilize both the transference and countertransference are her keen observational skills, and most importantly, self-awareness. The final story in this set of narratives is presented in two parts, **Chapter 36** and **Chapter 37**. It explores the emotional challenges inherent in caring for marginalized and vulnerable populations. This can be a crucible, both personally and professionally, for health care providers and ultimately challenge their commitment to being patient-centered. This is a narrative of courage, considerable self-reflection, and growth as a healer.

Chapter 38 describes how fatigue, exhaustion, and at worst, burnout, make clinicians susceptible to medical error. While the patient-doctor relationship may not be jeopardized, as this narrative indicates, it can result in suffering for the physician. This story challenges us to face our own vulnerability, fallibility and the need for forgiveness.

Chapter 39, albeit less dramatic than those that have preceded, is telling nonetheless. It illustrates the physician's sensitivity to the subtle nuances of the patient-doctor relationship that could easily have been dismissed or missed completely. But they were not, and as such, served to enhance the patient-doctor relationship.

The final story, **Chapter 40**, reveals how caring and compassion culminate in a healing process. The healing is bidirectional, as the relationship restores the capacity to be a healer for both the patient and the physician.

Narratives Illustrating Component IV:
Enhancing the Patient-Doctor Relationship

31 Unexplored Territory – Part 2

Joshua Shadd and Judith Belle Brown

It was early April, and the end of the school year was in sight. Marcus had excelled in his IT course and it appeared that this 19 year old had found his niche. Marcus wanted to finish well, but his nephroblastoma (Wilms' tumor, metastatic to lung and bone) was visibly progressing. His left neck and shoulder pain intensified, and he had new palpable lymphadenopathy in his neck. He had lost much of the mobility in his shoulder, and this was compromising his ability to play his bass guitar – his favorite pastime and form of escape. Dr. Boice had assumed Marcus's care when he had moved here to attend school almost nine months ago. They had faced some challenges as their therapeutic relationship evolved, but Dr. Boice felt a particular satisfaction in his part in Marcus's care and looked forward to their monthly appointments.

Two days before Dr. Boice was to leave for a week's vacation, Marcus called the clinic to say he was feeling dyspneic. Dr. Boice saw him that afternoon. For the first time, Marcus's girlfriend Angie attended clinic with him. Marcus was mildly tachycardic, but his physical examination was otherwise unchanged. He agreed to a chest X-ray but said he only wanted to know if he needed antibiotics or not. Marcus was blunt: "I can't handle any bad news today, doc."

The chest X-ray was, on the whole, reassuring. Marcus's metastases were growing slowly, but he had no evidence of new airspace disease. Dr. Boice chalked it up to an upper respiratory tract infection and the stress of impending exams. Dr. Boice booked a follow-up for after his vacation and instructed Marcus that if his breathing worsened in the meantime, he should go to the emergency room.

Dr. Boice returned from holiday to find his pager beeping on the bedside table, flashing the number of the emergency room. The next morning, Dr. Boice had barely walked through the office door when the clinic nurse told him Marcus's harrowing story. After his last appointment, Marcus had become progressively more dyspneic. When he finally presented to emergency, he had obvious stridor, and a repeat chest X-ray showed tracheal deviation. ("Was that visible on the X-ray I ordered?" Dr. Boice wondered as he listened.) An emergent CT scan demonstrated a soft tissue density occupying 95% of the cross-sectional area of his mid-trachea. Marcus's condition had been critical, and the emergency physician had paged Dr. Boice to ask what discussions they'd had regarding Marcus's goals of care.

When Dr. Boice heard this, he winced. Only his absence had saved him from having to admit that they had never talked about it. Marcus clearly told the emergency physician that he did not want intubation or tracheostomy. His family was summoned from their home town a few hours away. Fortunately, the thoracic surgeon was able to perform a partial resection via rigid bronchoscopy, and Marcus was discharged home two days later.

Marcus had dodged a bullet, and both he and Dr. Boice knew it. His next clinic visit had a different tone. Marcus talked about how frightened he had felt, but that he never once considered intubation. Marcus shook his head as he spoke, but there was conviction in his voice: "I've known for a long time that this disease is going to get me eventually. But I feel really lucky today. I've got my life back." At that visit, Dr. Boice and Marcus were finally able to have a discussion regarding goals of care and advance care planning. Marcus wanted his girlfriend, Angie, to be his substitute decision-maker. He still never mentioned his family.

That evening, with the final patient gone and last chart completed, Dr. Boice sat down at his desk, opened the top right-hand drawer, and pulled out a brown, leather-covered notebook. He called it his "Book of Musings." Dr. Boice certainly didn't think of himself as a writer, but he had always been in the habit of recording his thoughts on paper a couple times each week. Today, his thoughts came quickly.

April 19: Somebody once said that at the end of life, patients need a tour guide, not a fellow tourist. Tour guides anticipate; tourists react. The physician's role is to sensitively but honestly point out the bumps and potholes on the road ahead, helping patients and their families to avoid them if possible, or at least be prepared for them. I feel like I failed Marcus in this.

Should I have pushed him to have advance care planning discussions earlier? I knocked on that door regularly, but had not been welcomed. Should I have been more insistent? Would I have behaved differently with another patient?

Marcus is too young for what he is going through. Maybe that lends a different flavor to our relationship. Does Marcus, on some level, view me as a father figure? Is that part of why he never mentions his family? Do I, on some level, relish that role? Is this what they mean by "transference and countertransference"? Was that why I was so disappointed when I suspected Marcus was being untruthful regarding the lost pills? Is that part of why I've not asked him why he never mentions his family? What would I have learned if I had probed more deeply regarding his family?

Dr. Boice knew these questions were largely rhetorical, but he promised himself that he would bear them in mind at Marcus's next appointment. He could only hope that self-awareness and mindful practice would serve to enhance his ability to support Marcus and, ultimately, all of his future patients.

32 A Healing Presence

Joseph Lee, Judith Belle Brown and Tanya Thornton

I first met Bruno 15 years ago when I opened my practice. He was a 62-year-old university professor, married with two children. He was a gruff man, but with a quick smile and a penchant for telling jokes. He was an unapologetic chain-smoker, inhaling three packs a day. Bruno also enjoyed his single malt scotch neat, presented in a crystal tumbler. He had coarse facial features and was ever-ready to give his opinion on any subject, always eloquently executed in his thick European accent. His wife, Andrika, worried incessantly about Bruno's health. She always prepared a list of Bruno's symptoms before he came to see me. Bruno lovingly referred to her as his "house doctor," although she was not a physician. His daughter, however, *was* a physician – a subspecialist who had trained in the United States and subsequently became chief of department there. Bruno's son had followed his father's footsteps and was also on the faculty at the same university. Both children were very close to their parents and visited frequently.

Over time, Bruno developed a number of serious medical problems. The first was type 2 diabetes. Despite the diagnosis, Bruno remained unfazed. He was put on medications to control his blood sugar, but he made no attempt to change his lifestyle. Bruno continued to chain-smoke and did not lose weight or change his diet, much to his wife's and daughter's consternation. As our relationship evolved, his jokes became racier, which I interpreted as him being more comfortable with me.

It was only after developing angina that Bruno felt motivated to change his habits. With herculean effort, he quit smoking. Unfortunately, his angina worsened, and a coronary artery bypass graft was required. He did very well post-operatively and was able to enjoy his retirement and relish his reading. However, the greatest of Bruno's passions was writing, and as such, he embarked on the composition of his ninth book.

Then, Bruno developed kidney stones. He had a complicated course, eventually requiring stone fragmentation in a tertiary care center. During a recurrence of an episode of renal colic, investigations showed incidental enlargement of the retroperitoneal lymph nodes.

There was a delay in establishing the cause of the enlarged nodes, as the subsequent scans and needle biopsy failed to demonstrate the etiology. Meanwhile, Bruno began to suffer from weight loss, fatigue, malaise and back pain. Frustrated with waiting for further tests, Bruno's daughter arranged for him to fly to her hospital in the United States, where he had multiple scans and a repeat biopsy, which demonstrated metastatic cancer of the lung.

Upon his return from the United States, Bruno began chemotherapy. Although the prognosis for him was poor, the family insisted on treating him as aggressively as possible to extend his life. They were afraid to let him go. How could the fire and passion of this stellar man be allowed to fade and die?

The first two rounds of chemotherapy went poorly. The first resulted in hospitalization for a fever, the second in hospitalization for a diverticular abscess requiring surgical drainage. After these two rounds, I met with Bruno and his wife in my office. They sat solemnly together.

"I just don't understand why things aren't going well. He is strong, he came through his bypass with flying colors," Andrika vented, the frustration audible in her tremulous voice. "There must be another way to slow down the cancer," she pleaded in desperation.

"Well, there is a drug that may prevent the low cell counts, if Bruno pursues another round of chemo, but it's not always covered by private insurance," I began.

Bruno interrupted, shaking his head. "I'm not interested."

"What do you mean – of course you're interested!" Andrika retorted, the panic palpable in her voice.

Bruno turned to face his wife. "Listen, we know where this is going, we know there isn't a cure. I'm dying. I don't want to be sick for the little time I have left with you."

Andrika sobbed openly. She wasn't ready to give up, despite knowing that Bruno spoke the truth. He held her in silence. When they were ready, we explored together what Bruno valued, and what he wished for during the remainder of his life. "I want to continue writing my book. That damn chemo zapped all of my energy and concentration. I couldn't focus. I want to go home and be with my family." He paused. "I want to write while I still can." To that point in his care, Bruno had let his wife and daughter determine his treatment course. Things had changed. With her face blotchy from tears, Andrika solemnly agreed to her husband's wishes. Arrangements were made for palliation at home, and Bruno resumed working on his book.

The last time I saw Bruno was during a house call. He told me another joke. His wife and I had heard this one before, but we all laughed heartily nonetheless, particularly as Bruno delighted so much in the telling of the joke. We reflected on his remarkable life history, his many academic accomplishments and the passion that he held for his work. Although he did not subscribe to any organized religion, Bruno believed he had lived by certain principles, which he was proud to have followed. He valued honesty, respect and integrity – all of which personified his life. Bruno was proud of the many milestones he attained during his career, but he derived most of his fulfillment in his loving marriage and his children's achievements.

Bruno's only regret was that he was too weak to finish writing the very last chapter of his book. We discussed this and had a similar viewpoint – that one would want to live life such that there would always be something not quite done, something one was still wishing to accomplish.

Bruno passed away peacefully a few days later.

Despite Bruno's daughter's earlier disillusionment with her father's care, she came to understand that what her father needed and yearned for was an advocate who heard his heart's desires, understood his losses and actively cared to the end. In essence, a physician, or more accurately, a therapeutic relationship, that empowered him and re-established his control over the suffering. I, as his family physician, assumed the role of advocate and facilitated communication between Bruno and his family. In the end, I was powerless at healing Bruno's body but was able to foster an emotional healing more powerful, one that made Bruno whole again. Bruno's losses were restored, which enabled him to reconnect with the passions that had driven his life and eased his dying.

I will always remember Bruno. He had lived life with unrestrained enthusiasm and energy. I admired his sharp intellect and the unwavering principles that guided his life. And I will miss his jokes, and his love of telling them. They remarkably served as the bond that sealed our patient-doctor relationship.

33 A Familiar Kiss Goodbye

Eric Wong and Tanya Thornton

Beep-beep-beep. Beep-beep-beep. My pager displayed the extension of the emergency room. "*Damn it!*" I thought. "*It's not like I'm not busy enough already ... another admission from the emerg.*" I was frustrated. It was the fourth day of my seven-day workweek as a hospitalist locum, and I was already tired from caring for the 32 patients on the medical ward. After my emotions settled, I reluctantly put the pen in my shirt pocket and slapped shut my patient's chart. "*I'll come back to it later ... I've got no choice,*" I concluded.

I spoke with the emergency physician, who explained that an elderly woman, age 75, had likely suffered a stroke and was having difficulty communicating. My weary legs sauntered through the emergency room, its cacophony of noise and beeps awakening my senses.

I approached room two, where my new admission – Mai Jung – lay. I just wanted to get this done and finish rounds on the rest of my patients. As I knocked on the door, I took a peek inside. Mai Jung was lying peacefully on the stretcher, her eyes closed. A sensation of panic thundered through my body, as it crossed my mind that perhaps her stroke had worsened and caused her to become unconscious. I quickened to the side of the bed and called out her name loudly and repeatedly. Finally she answered on my third attempt and looked straight at me with glimmering eyes and a big smile.

After a few brief questions, it was obvious that Mai Jung had difficulty comprehending what I was saying, and her words were mumbled. A CT scan of Mai Jung's brain showed changes consistent with an early stroke. It was in an area of the brain that would result in comprehension and speech difficulties. I was relieved to discover that Mai Jung had been a previously healthy woman, which meant that the admission process would not be lengthy.

As I said goodbye to Mai Jung and was walking out of her room, I was stopped by a middle-aged woman. "Are you the doctor who's going to be taking care of my mom, Mai Jung? I'm Nora, her daughter."

I looked at her and knew she was frightened. Her eyes were about to overflow with tears, and her voice was shaky. I replied, "Yes," and proceeded to give Nora a summary of her mother's medical condition. I reassured her that based on the current findings, her mother had suffered a small stroke but had a good chance of recovery. "However, we need to monitor her for a few days and do some more tests," I explained. Despite my best efforts, Nora was not reassured, but as I had other patients to attend to, she reluctantly released me from her slew of questions. As she turned her back towards me, she headed over to Mai Jung, kissed her on the forehead, held her hand in hers, and began weeping quietly while sitting on a chair beside Mai Jung's bed. Mai Jung seemed indifferent, but the quivering of her lips told me that she was trying to say something.

When I made my rounds the next morning, I entered Mai Jung's room only to find someone whom I could not quite recognize. It was a sunny day, and the warm light of the morning sun cast soft shadows over the face of the woman who sat in the tacky orange armchair that was awkwardly placed in the corner of the room. The woman was elegantly dressed in a white blouse and navy blue trousers. You could tell that she had paid special attention to her hair, because her brunette curls looked organized and bouncy. As I regained my composure, I realized that red lipstick painted her smiling face and she was staring straight into my eyes with a kindness that felt only too familiar. "Good morning, doctor," Mai Jung said with perfect articulation and intonation. "I am feeling much better today. Thank you for seeing me yesterday."

My heart jumped at Mai Jung's remarkable, speedy recovery. Not everyone who has a stroke recovers so quickly and seemingly without residual deficits. I chatted briefly with Mai Jung about her condition and reassured her that she would only need to stay a few days for further tests. I wanted to speak with her more, perhaps because of that familiar kindness I felt.

Later that day, I received a phone call from Nora inquiring about Mai Jung's condition. I reassured Nora that her mother was recovering quite well and would be discharged soon. However, an awkward silence followed, rather than the one which I expected to be filled with a joyous response. Instead, as the silence broke, I realized that Nora was crying. "I'm so glad," Nora said with a tremor in her voice, "She's the best person I know in this world."

As I visited Mai Jung over the next few days, I came to know her better. She grew up on a farm and was married to her husband for 40 years before he had passed away a few years back. Mai Jung had been living by herself since that time and was completely independent. She maintained close contact with her children. I learned a bit more about Mai Jung's life story each day as the topic of conversation gradually evolved from medical updates to much more enjoyable exchanges about our lives. Mai Jung had such a wonderful way of telling her simple stories that it made me feel like I was experiencing them first-hand.

Mai Jung's investigations concluded uneventfully, and the day came when she was about to leave the hospital. Nora was present and had invited her mother to stay with her for a few weeks before Mai Jung returned to her own home. The setting sun shed its golden colors in the room and beauti-fied everything that was in it. Even the tacky orange armchair now seemed harmonic with the rest of the room. Yet the air in the room was solemn, and there was this fog over my heart that felt somehow suffocating. As I stepped into the room, I could sense the difference – the feeling that this room would never imprint the same impression on me again.

I was greeted with warm smiles from both mother and daughter. Nora quickly began to thank me for the care that I had given her mom. For some-one who had always been uncomfortable being the center of attention, I simply replied with the truth, "Mai Jung's body healed itself. I just super-vised the process."

I knew the time for goodbye was near. I knelt down in front of Mai Jung, who was sitting on the side of her bed, packed and ready. I placed my hand on top of her knee and said without hesitation, "It has been wonderful to have known you, Mai Jung. I wish you all the best."

She looked at me in the eyes again, and once more, I felt that familiar-ity that I was unable to explain. Her eyes had changed. The added moisture made them glitter even more. As I was about to shake her hand, she took me in her arms and planted a kiss on my cheek. "Thank you," she whispered. As much as my stomach started to turn, and my heart began to swell, I half-consciously returned Mai Jung's gesture by placing a kiss on her cheek. It was the first kiss I had ever given to a patient.

All of a sudden, I understood. I understood that feeling of familiarity with Mai Jung. Mai Jung had become more than my patient. As I hugged this ever-loving mother, I realized that she had become the image of my grandmother who had passed away suddenly five years ago. My grandma had a very special place in my heart. She was what mattered most in my world as a child and young adolescent, and I missed her terribly. When she died, I never had a chance to kiss her goodbye, until now.

34 A Gift Offered – a Gift Received

Jeff Sisler and Judith Belle Brown

Nettie was a tense woman in her early 70s with a lined face, thick glasses in brown frames and hair blacker than her years would allow. I had known her for three years, and they had been eventful ones. A colonoscopy a year ago had resulted in surgery for bowel cancer. Sedatives had become a regular feature of her life since her cancer, and we'd had many a go-nowhere discussion about "finding other ways to cope." She and her husband, Frank, had two children, one of whom, Roberta, had died tragically in the hospital a month previous at the age of 47. Roberta's life and her relationship with her family had been tumultuous. Nettie's voice had always dropped to a whisper when Roberta became the topic of conversation.

Our visit that day was to check on how Nettie was managing her profound grief following Roberta's death. It was an odd visit. She avoided eye contact, appearing nervous and distracted. Her answers to my questions were evasive and didn't invite me in any further. Settling for the fact that she was still socializing and that her use of sedatives had decreased, I acknowledged how she was doing and rose to my feet. "Wait!" Nettie said with alarm. "I have something for you." She dug into the battered brown purse she had tucked under the chair and pulled out a white envelope. "This is for you," she said, her eyes filling with tears. Nettie's voice shook. "It meant so much to know you were helping out Roberta in the hospital and talking to Frank and me. It meant so much to us." I opened up the envelope and met the eyes of Robert Borden, who stared back at me impassively. One hundred Canadian dollars! How could she? Disbelief and shock sent my mind racing.

Roberta was diagnosed with a bipolar disorder in her 30s and had been in and out of the hospital, jobs and relationships ever since. What I knew of her I had learned from Nettie and from my clinic partner, who was Roberta's family doctor. Roberta was a worry for both of them. Four months ago she had arrived in the emergency room on a Saturday evening, after her son found her lying in a confused state on the floor of her apartment. Roberta told the emergency physician that she had felt her legs crumble underneath her while walking to the bathroom. She had spent the whole day on the floor, unable to crawl to a phone. In the hospital, she was remote and unconcerned, a bit dehydrated, and neither of her legs could move. She spent that night in the observation unit and was given intravenous fluids and the diagnosis of depression and paraplegia.

I reviewed Roberta that next Sunday morning. The picture was both unusual and interesting. She had no movement in her legs and very little in her feet. Both legs appeared numb, and her reflexes were somewhat diminished. Her blood tests were all reasonable. Roberta remained distant and hard to engage in conversation. She admitted to feeling quite depressed for the last several weeks and described having a lot of muscle pain in her back and hips. None of this was entirely new. Roberta then made the curious remark that her landlord had also become paralyzed the year before and had had to stop working. I plowed through her old chart, all three volumes, full of stories of anxiety, somatic preoccupation, electroconvulsive therapy, family turmoil and a changing cast of psychiatric medications. Nonetheless, Roberta certainly couldn't move her legs and it became clear she couldn't urinate on her own either. Back X-rays were ordered and were interpreted as normal, although their quality was somewhat poor. Puzzled, I made the decision to ask neurology to see her that day.

Neurologic examinations are notorious for their poor consistency, and it seemed that everyone who examined Roberta got a slightly different picture. We did agree, though, that she could barely move her legs and that they seemed quite numb. Too numb in fact – the neurologist assessed the level of sensory loss in her mid-back, but found her reflexes normal. One thing was clear – the pattern wasn't consistent with a spinal cord injury, and Roberta was a woman with a past. This was the first conversion disorder I had seen. I handed Roberta's care over to my partner, her family physician, the next day with the excitement of having witnessed something strange and remarkable.

On the ward, Roberta's legs did seem to improve slowly, but she became increasingly concerned at the slow pace of her recovery. I would speak to her on weekends when I was on call and talk with Nettie and Frank when I ran into them at the hospital. We agreed it was terribly frustrating and a most unusual kind of problem. But perhaps not so unusual, given all that they had already been through with Roberta.

A new neurology resident examined Roberta. He was puzzled by her ongoing symptoms and upon hearing her growing frustration suggested a CT scan be ordered. So it was three weeks after Roberta's admission, after everything from physiotherapy to psychiatry, from medication to abreaction had been tried to convince her psyche to release its prisoners, when Roberta had the CT scan. It revealed not only the complete collapse of her fourth thoracic vertebra but also the tumors in her pelvis and also hinted at the mass in her pancreas. This was perhaps the real culprit of her precarious situation. Roberta received some dexamethasone in an attempt to reduce the swelling and pressure on her spinal cord. It didn't help. Neither did the radiotherapy. Two months later, she died, paralyzed, hallucinating, with her family at her bedside.

You'll understand now why Robert Borden's eyes unnerved me so and why I felt a sense of horror. Nettie's eyes were moist as she firmly stated again: "This is for you, to thank you for all you did for Roberta and how you helped." I felt like shouting, *"Don't you realize this was the most awful mistake I've ever been part of? And you're giving me money?"*

But instead of confession, I responded with careful formality. "Oh, Nettie, I couldn't possibly accept such a generous gift. It just wouldn't be right." "Please," she said, making eye contact for the first time, "You deserve it."

A gift offered.

A gift bearing another gift – one of healing for a doctor with a troubled conscience.

A gift received.

35 A Misalignment Offers Understanding

Lemmese Al-Watban and Judith Belle Brown

Zack, age 40, was a new patient on my roster. When I first met him, I was impressed by his physical presence. He was a towering, large-boned man, standing at well over six feet tall and weighing about 200 pounds. But in contrast, his demeanor was that of a timid and bashful individual. The juxtaposition of his presentation baffled me – the dissonance was somehow unsettling, but I could not comprehend why I felt this way.

Zack had come to see me because he was interested in trying a new antidepressant. "I saw this new drug for depression advertised on television, and I would like to try it out," Zack asked cautiously. Further questioning revealed that his request had been triggered after a two-month relationship had ended with his female friend, Samantha. Zack painfully described how he was feeling, "When I am alone, well I just feel empty." His primary worry was that the depression he had experienced during and after his divorce was returning.

Zack's concerns were focused on his feelings of being alone and isolated. He was very emotional when he stated that his greatest fear might become a reality. "Lena, my ex-wife, was right, I will always be alone without her," Zack stated despairingly.

Zack's chart revealed that he had a past history of mild depression that had lasted for several years. He had been treated with antidepressants and had seen a therapist regularly. Zack believed his depression was the consequence of his 15-year abusive marriage. After Zack's divorce two years ago, his mood improved dramatically and he was slowly weaned off of his antidepressants. He continued to meet with his therapist weekly, up until six months ago, when they decided to space the visits out to once a month.

"I usually would talk to Shelley, my therapist, about my week, but now I don't see her until the end of the month," Zack anxiously explained. The recent change in his usual counseling schedule from once a week to once a month was also contributing to his loneliness and reflected another loss for Zack. In addition, Zack expressed concern about not having any family or friends to talk to about his concerns, let alone basic human interactions regarding daily experiences of living. He conceded that he did not know how to make friends. "My ex-wife never allowed me to have friends," he expressed in a desolate tone.

Zack demonstrated both anguish about how his ex-wife had abused him, as well as disappointment with himself for letting it go on for so long. "Lena ruined my life! I am too old to start all over," Zack stated with despair. He was terrified of once again spiraling into a depression and feared regressing into his old dietary habits. "I need to keep up with my exercise and remind myself that I am doing this for me," Zack explained with exasperation. Finally, Zack feared his newfound sense of control over his life would be lost. What ultimately frightened Zack was the mere thought that his ex-wife might be right: "Maybe I am just a loser."

Zack had been diagnosed with type 2 diabetes six years ago. He was convinced the onset of his diabetes was a direct result of his abusive marriage. "I was always depressed and comforted myself with food," he explained. After his divorce Zack lost 30 pounds, was exercising regularly and had maintained well-controlled blood sugars. However, Zack had noticed an increase in his appetite and had been finding it difficult to maintain a diabetic diet, especially when he was home alone, as he found that he craved "comfort food."

Since his divorce, Zack had experienced a dramatic change in his life, yet he ruminated about his relationship with Lena. He had been attracted to her strong personality and good looks, but during their entire marriage Lena had been abusive both verbally and physically. Zack's independence had been rapidly diminished. Lena demanded that he quit his job and work at her hardware store. He was not allowed to have friends or go out on his own without Lena at his side. She even controlled what he would wear, eat and drink. "I wasn't allowed to think for myself," Zack painfully explained.

With the support of his therapist, Zack had extricated himself from his marriage. While Zack was exuberant to be free from Lena's controlling and abusive ways, he was notably unsure about how to move forward with his life. "I feel like I have lost my identity and I no longer know how to live for myself," he said with a profound sadness.

Soon after I assumed Zack's care, he began making multiple visits to the office within a short period of time for follow-up of his well-controlled diabetes. He always started our conversations with an apology for wasting my time and constantly asked me to help him make day-to-day decisions. "Doctor, please tell me what to do," Zack would ask in a pleading tone.

I began to wonder if Zack's behavior suggested some transference issues. I questioned whether my role as his doctor might have been a bit hazy to Zack. On several occasions I wondered, "*Did Zack consider me more as a friend or even as a substitute decision-maker, similar to his ex-wife?*"

I also began to reflect on whether there may have been some countertransference on my behalf. I had been taken aback by the incongruity between his appearance and his demeanor. His frequent and unnecessary visits made me uncomfortable. I began to wonder if he had taken a personal interest in me. In addition, I was concerned that perhaps my initial detached stance had contributed to a perception, on Zack's behalf, that my personality was similar to his ex-wife's. *"Was I becoming a replacement for his need for codependency?"* I pondered.

After gaining a greater awareness of the complex dynamic of our patient-doctor relationship, I tried to put more effort into encouraging Zack to increase his network of acquaintances. We had no difficulty on reaching common ground in identifying Zack's medical problems and the goals of treatment. But I worried that Zack often acquiesced to my recommendations. It remained a challenge to keep our roles clear as Zack remained passive and quick to agree with me. It was important to reinforce my role as his doctor and not as his substitute wife.

When patients have experienced an abusive relationship, like Zack, it is important for the physician to be attuned to nuances in the patient-doctor relationship. It is also imperative to maintain an equal balance of power in the relationship. The focus should be on empowering the patient and avoiding any behavior that may mimic the past relationship with the abusive partner. For example, providing resources and guidance to increase Zack's self-confidence and social networks were important in helping him re-establish his identity.

Understanding how the patient's transference may be an unconscious attempt to replicate the past relationship can be a critical source of information. In the relationship with Zack, his transference illuminated his strong need for dependency and thus guided my therapeutic role of giving him back the power and independence he needed in his life.

Physician self-awareness is also essential in order to attend to potential countertransference issues that can impede the therapeutic relationship. Again, in reflecting on the relationship with Zack, I realized that to have responded to his neediness would have been a disservice to his ultimate goal of being an independent and autonomous individual.

In conclusion, transference and countertransference are not negative or adverse aspects of the patient-doctor relationship if they are addressed accordingly. They can, in fact, offer important information regarding how past relationships influence and dictate current interactions. This knowledge is invaluable in caring for patients. Understanding our own countertransference also offers an unlimited window into our role as healers. Self-awareness, coupled with mindfulness, is the key.

Judith Belle Brown and Susan Woolhouse

Caring for vulnerable populations involves successes and failures – joys and sorrows. Caring can be, from the perspective of a clinician, both a personal and professional crucible. This crucible can be labeled as compassion fatigue, vicarious trauma or burnout. Regardless of the label, the following experiences of a health care provider are both powerful and poignant.

"Chin up, shoulders back, body erect, "I kept saying to myself, a mantra of sorts, as I entered the drop-in center for homeless, drug-using women. I had been gone for a few months and vowed upon my return that I would never, never trudge back in, slumped-over, ready to do battle. I had begun at the center over one year ago on a crusade. My vision of empowering these marginalized women – getting them clean, out of the sex trade, housed and safe from the chaos and violence that permeated their lives – went up in flames. And so did I.

Fresh out of training, I had come bearing an armamentarium of best practices, health promotion strategies, and of course, a belief in patient-centered care. Despite my noble efforts to save these vulnerable women from what I perceived to be their tragic existence, I began to wonder if some of my well-intentioned tactics were drawing them deeper into their dark worlds. I thought I could rescue women, but in reality, I had become paternalistic, controlling and more judgmental. Two women in particular forced me to reconsider my role as their family physician.

Bea, aged 37, had been on the street for 20 years. She was an active crack user and had multiple complications of AIDS. Bea rarely came to the center, but on this occasion she presented to have the sutures in her skull removed. The details of the story were scant, but a violent altercation over a drug deal "gone bad" had left Bea with a severe head wound requiring 30 stitches. This was not the first time she had been a victim of violence – her scarred body was proof. As I carefully attended to her wound, I implored Bea to consider going to a women's shelter where she would be safe and also to come to the center more often.

"Ain't got time, doc," she had replied in a blunt manner and fell silent for the remainder of the procedure, despite my constant barrage of questions and requests to help her. I did not know this would be the last time I would see Bea.

It was heartbreaking to bear witness to someone who I thought was destroying herself and appeared to be unable to change her situation. I just didn't know if I could go on seeing women travelling down such a painful path that would ultimately result in death. Intellectually, I knew death for vulnerable women using illicit drugs was often premature and violent. But I worried about how devastating and emotionally draining it would be to have one of the women I cared for become another statistic on the news – brutally murdered. I didn't know if I had the strength or the stamina to listen to the news on the morning radio and hear about another sex trade worker being killed, or see the headlines splashed across the front page of the newspaper.

Then what I feared most happened. Bea was in the news – she was one of those statistics. The headline read: "Small businessmen upset about effect of another shooting in the area – addict and prostitute shot." Bea had been shot in the chest and slowly bled out in a cold, dark alley – alone. Just as Bea was stigmatized and undervalued in her life, the media further marginalized her in her death by focusing on the economic impact of her murder. My heart was gutted, my guilt overwhelming. I had failed to keep Bea safe from harm.

My other patient was Carla. In contrast to Bea, this 26–year-old woman frequently attended the center with a multitude of physical, emotional or social crises. While her visits were brief, they were always intense. Carla was also homeless and a sex trade worker. She was often forced into extraordinarily risky situations in order to secure drugs for her abusive partner or to pay for a safe place to sleep for the night. Carla's male partner was often in and out of jail. When he was in jail, there was a sense of relief, but when he was released, the violent beatings would start again.

With a steely surge of courage, Carla was able to break away from this torturous relationship. One day Carla bounced into the center announcing that she was pregnant. "I'm going to get off the dope," she declared, and with eager anticipation said, "I want a kid to love and love me back." Carla struggled to stop using drugs throughout her pregnancy.

I wasn't sure what I found more heartbreaking – the potential harm that was being done to Carla's fetus through her drug use or the fact that getting pregnant was the only strategy she had to feel loved and wanted in this world. Despite these mixed feelings, I meticulously prepared a schedule for Carla's prenatal care. Her visits were rare and sporadic, and Carla struggled to follow my recommendations. During her second trimester, Carla came crashing into the center. "I ain't feeling the baby no more!" she wailed. Her partner had once again re-entered Carla's life and his systematic and severe beatings of Carla had escalated. The end result – her baby was dead. The depth of her shame was bottomless and unrelenting – the shame of being homeless, the shame of being a sex trade worker, the shame of being a drug user, the shame of being abused, and ultimately, the shame of failing to safeguard her unborn child.

I also felt shame. Shame for the intense anger that raged inside me towards Carla, her abusive partner, the health care system, society's failure to provide adequate supports for women like Carla, and finally, at myself. I had failed to keep Carla and her fetus safe from harm. My despair was overwhelming.

Judith Belle Brown and Susan Woolhouse

After Bea's horrific death and Carla's tragic loss, I came to realize I was rapidly "flaming out." Somewhat in disbelief, I had a dawning awareness that perhaps I was exhibiting the classic symptoms of burnout. I was emotionally exhausted and overwhelmed by the burden of caring for this vulnerable population. In my work at the center I had started going through the day like an "automaton." And my sense of personal accomplishment was radically diminished. Yes, I was burning out.

So I took a leave of absence from the center. Perhaps I was just not cut out for this job. I wasn't sure. What I did know was that how I had been approaching my work with these women, who were trapped in the vortex of their chaotic lives, was not working. The violence was contagious, the despair palpable. If I was to care and to value these vulnerable women as worthwhile human beings, regardless of their actions or life choices, I had to learn a new way to listen to and to understand their stories of pain. Instead of my crusade to rescue them, I had to be present for them.

By trying to rescue these women, I had become paternalistic and less patient-centered. I was missing out on the wonderful relationships that I had with my patients, a group of incredible women. I had forgotten to celebrate the victories that we able to achieve together. When I got caught up in the chaos of my patients' lives, I had failed to see these women for the strong, resilient and courageous people that they were. Wasn't it amazing that Carla had the courage to leave her partner, even that one time? How could I forget the wonderful volunteer work that Bea did with other sex workers in the center? She used to distribute condoms to sex workers who didn't feel comfortable coming into our center. And what a sense of humor she had! How she could make me laugh! My own burnout was taking the joy out of my job.

During my time away I did some serious reflection and received sage counsel from several wise mentors. I was returning with new strategies – well actually, a new way of being. I had left my crusade behind. I now appreciated both the rewards and the challenges provided by my work.

Carolyn was at the top of the patient list my first day back. Like so many of the other women I had seen in the past, her story was a tragic one. She had apparently been living on the streets on and off since adolescence and had been living with HIV and chronic hepatitis C for over five years. She had been told she was "bipolar" by a doctor as a teenager but could not elaborate further. Her use of crack cocaine was a way to "numb" her feelings and help her cope with the daily struggles that come with street life. Apparently, staff at the drop-in had been bugging her for so long to "get her HIV checked out" that she finally "gave in." Her only concern that day was pain in her mouth. She was unable to recall the last time she had her HIV blood work done but told me that her "counts were really low." On examination, she showed signs of oral candidiasis (secondary to the HIV). In contrast to her thin and cachectic body, her eyes darted quickly around the room, avoiding eye contact with me, and she exhibited fidgety movements. She looked like she wanted to crawl out of her skin. The more questions I asked, the more restless she became.

After about five minutes, Carolyn had reached her limit. I paused for a moment, and then quickly summarized, "Carolyn, it looks like we should wrap things up for today. For not having seen a doctor in so long, you sure did a great job today putting up with all these questions. Here is a medication that will help with the mouth pain. Will you come see me again next week to tell me if the medication worked? Maybe you could think of some other things you want to talk about?" Carolyn shrugged her shoulders and stated in a somewhat dismissive tone, "Okay. I'll think about it." Then as she walked out the door, she turned, smiled slightly and said: "Hey, they were right – you're not so bad."

I think I was finally getting it. Now my overall objective was to develop a therapeutic relationship with these women. I had modified my expectations – the celebration now is when they come back. It was crucial to establish trust and ensure that these women felt secure and respected. I had also come to understand how being nonjudgmental would be important during this engagement phase. "Your job is to make women feel welcome," one mentor told me, "and they also need to know that people recognize, despite their drug problems and other issues, they're okay people." I needed to accept my patients at face value. And while I might not endorse their lifestyles, I would still be accepting of these women. They were human beings who deserved to be cared for and respected.

I knew there would be times when the women would test me to ensure that the center was a safe place to receive their health care. Many of the women had very negative experiences with the health care system, so I would need to show them that I was going to "hang in there." By "meeting them where they're at" and not abandoning them, I would gain their trust – trust being the core foundation of our relationship. But I would go slowly, be present, nonjudgmental and flexible. It would be hard not to get caught up in the chaos and the roller-coaster rides, but I was committed to trying.

In the past I had experienced the emotional impact of witnessing the overwhelming tragedies experienced by my former patients. I had been traumatized by their chaos, pain, loss and even death. My patients' losses became my losses. I hoped that my new approach would temper this pain and would assist me in remaining present. Now, I feel more able to celebrate the strong and meaningful relationships I have with these women. I will try to support my patients to celebrate successes, accept failures without judgment, savor the moments of joy, and respond to sorrow with compassion.

38 An Urgent Request – a Delayed Response

Judith Belle Brown, W. Wayne Weston and Moira Stewart

Late Saturday evening, I entered my home office to discover my beeper violently vibrating across my desk. I was surprised, as I wasn't on call and had carefully handed over my patients to enjoy a well-needed weekend of relaxation. It had been a hectic few weeks with several critically ill patients and a serious flu epidemic to contend with. I was exhausted and sorely in need of rest.

I grabbed my beeper with frustration to discover 10 messages from the answering service stating: "Urgent – Please Reply ASAP." Upon calling the service, the switchboard operator indicated that the daughters of one of my elderly patients had contacted the answering service 40 times in the last eight hours. I was flabbergasted! What was going on? Why hadn't the physician on call been notified? The short answer to my questions was that my patient's daughters flatly refused to speak to anyone but me. The normally calm and reserved switchboard operator strongly requested I contact them as soon as possible. Her exasperation was palpable.

Reluctantly, and with some degree of resentment, I called the number she had given me. When I identified myself the voice on the other end of the telephone demanded: "Where have you been? You have been my mother's doctor the last four years, she is your responsibility! You must admit her to hospital immediately!"

The speaker's voice sounded vaguely familiar, and I quickly recognized it to be Mrs. Van de Root's daughter, Erin, whom I had met a couple of times. Startled by her aggressive stance, I quickly inquired about her mother's status. "Well we took her for a long walk today and afterwards she seemed very unsteady. We think you should admit her to hospital to be assessed!" she stated adamantly. Somewhat taken aback, I asked to speak to my patient, 82-year-old Mrs. Amelia Van de Root. Sounding somewhat embarrassed, Mrs. Van de Root stated: "I am fine. My two daughters are visiting and are just worried about me. You know getting old is just not fun, but I am okay." Not fully reassured by my frail and aging patient, I contacted the nursing staff at the retirement home where Mrs. Van de Root had resided since becoming a widow two years ago. The nurse reassured me that they had not noted any significant changes in her recent health status. Based on this information, I contacted Mrs. Van de Root's daughters indicating I would assess their mother the next morning at 8 a.m. While not pleased with this conclusion, they acquiesced. I went to bed feeling resentful and depleted – again.

The next morning I arose, went for a short run and then drove over to the retirement home, once again feeling both reluctant and somewhat resentful. When I entered her well-appointed suite at the residence, I found Mrs. Van de Root sitting in a chair at her kitchen table, alert, dressed and in no distress. Her two daughters were just finishing breakfast with their mother. Mrs. Van de Root greeted me warmly. "So good of you, doctor, to visit on such a blustery November day – and a Sunday nonetheless. Please come in, come in!" The two daughters glared at me – their anger was overt yet unspoken in the presence of their mother.

Certainly Mrs. Van de Root had gradually been getting frailer over the last four years. She came to the office every two months, mainly for blood pressure checks and reassurance. She had bilateral macular degeneration and her vision was very poor. She was able to watch television and could read the newspaper with a magnifying glass. Her only medications were Enalapril 5 mg daily and ASA 81 mg daily. Her last weight taken in the office was 105 lbs.

When I asked Mrs. Van de Root how she was feeling, she replied that she was getting weaker and more unsteady on her feet. She had had several falls in her living room. Otherwise the review of systems was negative. Her physical exam revealed a heart rate of 70 beats per minute, in regular rhythm, a blood pressure of 130/85, and a chest that was clear to auscultations. Her abdomen was soft, with no organomegaly. Her pupils were equal and reactive; the cranial nerves were intact. She could move all her limbs, and power was equal on both sides. Her skin showed no obvious bruises.

On the basis of this assessment, I concluded she was becoming frailer, but there was no acute disease process going on and no need for a hospital admission. After conferring with the patient, the nursing supervisor at her place of residence and her two daughters, we decided on the following plan. First, nursing care would come in daily and report to me as required. Second, I would request a geriatric consultation to be done at the residence on a non-urgent basis, with a view that the patient required additional care.

Mrs. Van de Root's daughters' anger subsided to some extent, and they left the next day, returning to their homes almost 125 miles away. I did not hear from the nursing staff until a week later.

During the night, the nursing staff at Mrs. Van de Root's residence had become very concerned about her increasing weakness and complaint of a headache over the last week. She was taken to the hospital by ambulance, and the emergency physician admitted Mrs. Van de Root with a diagnosis of a transient ischemic attack. There had been no neurological signs upon examination, and a CT of the head was ordered for the next morning.

Neurology was consulted and reviewed the CT scan of her head, which revealed a large, frontal subdural fluid collection. Mrs. Van de Root was taken to surgery, where two burr holes were performed. Over 250 mLs of yellow fluid were drained, indicating there had been a chronic subdural hematoma. Post-operatively, her recovery was precarious, but over time she recovered most of her function. Remarkably, her mental faculties remained intact, and she was able to ambulate with the aid of a walker. Most importantly, Mrs. Van de Root's spirits improved, and her zest for life returned.

But my zest for clinical practice was still dampened. I had failed my patient. *How had I missed this diagnosis of a subdural hematoma? Had I been distracted by my own fatigue and frustration? The patient's daughters' persistence and anger had been annoying, but had it seriously detracted me from my ability to attentively listen to my patient's story? Had it obstructed my capacity as a clinician to pick up on the subtle clues of her subdural hematoma? Perhaps I was too absorbed in my own needs for physical and emotional respite from the seemingly never-ending demands of my clinical practice in recent years. On the other hand, the angry and demanding behavior of my patient's daughters may have made me both defensive and equally acrimonious. But how had I missed the essential signs – increasing falls in her suite at the retirement residence, and the onset of headaches in the preceding weeks – I had not asked about headaches, and my patient had not offered this information. Nonetheless, it was my responsibility to inquire.*

To this day I struggle with not fully understanding all that happened in those few days. Perhaps if I had listened more attentively and had not been distracted by the extraneous noise of others, both of family and of caregivers, then perhaps I could have prevented this assault on my patient's life and on my psyche. Then again … perhaps I could not.

39 The Patient-Physician Relationship over Time

Bridget L. Ryan

Like all good relationships, the patient-physician relationship can grow and improve over time. It may not always start out well, even with the best of intentions. But when both the patient and the physician give each other the benefit of the doubt and demonstrate respect for one another, the relationship can become a powerful one.

Kathleen, a vibrant, healthy 82 year old, was grieving the death of Al, her husband of 60 years. Fiercely independent, she rarely took time for her own health care and was not one to "bother the doctor" for herself. Kathleen had devoted her life to caring for others, including her mother-in-law, her three children, her mother and most recently, her husband, who had been diagnosed with cancer of the liver two years prior.

Dr. Stafford had been the couple's doctor since they moved to Preston 10 years ago to be closer to one of their sons and his family. Initially, Kathleen was uncertain how she felt about Dr. Stafford, comparing him unfavorably to their previous family doctor in Oakdale. One of their initial conversations concerned the propranolol Kathleen was taking for atypical angina. Dr. Stafford believed the dose was so small as to not be therapeutic and instructed her to discontinue the medication and return to the office in one week. They discussed this plan, and Kathleen reluctantly agreed. But as she left the office she was unconvinced that this was a good idea.

Her previous doctor had prescribed the propranolol for her angina, and she had absolute confidence in his medical care. Kathleen returned in a week complaining of shortness of breath, which she had not had in years. Dr. Stafford put her back on the same low dose of propranolol. In subsequent visits over the years, Dr. Stafford would sometimes mention this encounter and say, "Well we don't want to change the propranolol. It works well for you." Kathleen, although initially angry that Dr. Stafford had challenged her previous doctor's management plan, began to appreciate Dr. Stafford's style, and his forthrightness in admitting that his initial plan for her regarding the management of her angina had not been the most effective.

Over the years, and particularly through her husband's difficult illness, Kathleen and Dr. Stafford had forged a good relationship based on mutual respect for one another's views. Dr. Stafford visited Kathleen and her husband at home when Al was no longer able to visit the office. The first time Kathleen visited the office after Al's death – for a routine visit to refill prescriptions – Dr. Stafford spent a good deal of time with Kathleen just chatting: about Al, about Kathleen not sleeping well and her loss of weight, and the enormity of her grief.

Kathleen told Dr. Stafford how completely lost she felt. "My children and their families are very good to me, but I just miss Al so much. I'm just lost without him."

Dr. Stafford responded, "Of course, Kathleen. But you are doing just fine – it's only been a couple of months. Over the years, I saw how close you and Al were. You had a wonderful marriage. Don't let anyone tell you how long to grieve. Just take your time and look after yourself."

Kathleen felt empowered by Dr. Stafford's appreciation of the depth of her grief. Later, when a friend suggested that she needed to get on with life and not sit at home wallowing, she answered, "I am getting out a bit. My doctor said that everyone grieves in their own way. And that I should take my time and not feel rushed."

Three months later, when she returned to the office for her prescription renewals, Dr. Stafford affectionately greeted her with, "I thought I told you not to be a stranger!" Knowing that Kathleen was unlikely to visit "just to talk," he took this opportunity to ask her how things were going. While chatting, he noticed a concerning spot on her cheek. Given that Kathleen had been treated for skin cancer five years ago, Dr. Stafford indicated that he would like her to see someone about having the spot removed. "I don't think it is anything life-threatening, but I do think you should have it removed."

Kathleen hesitated for a moment, then said, "You know, doctor, I really don't want to go back to the Cancer Clinic right now. I spent so much time there with Al, and I don't think I can do that."

Dr. Stafford immediately responded, "Absolutely. No, I don't want you to go there right now either. I was thinking I would send you to a dermatologist to have it removed."

"Oh," sighed Kathleen with apparent relief, "that's fine then. I will do that."

Dr. Stafford continued talking with Kathleen. "You are looking a lot better than last time, Kathleen. I'm pleased to see that your weight has stabilized. You're still not very heavy, but that's okay – that's healthier. I wish all my patients were like that!"

"I'm sleeping better too," offered Kathleen.

Dr. Stafford inquired about how Kathleen was getting around.

"Oh, I take taxis to come here," she answered.

He further explored, "And you're getting out of the apartment sometimes?"

Proudly Kathleen explained, "Oh, absolutely – I get out with my sons and my next-door neighbors, and I go to church on Sunday."

"Good, I'm pleased to hear that, Kathleen," replied Dr. Stafford.

As Kathleen prepared to leave, Dr. Stafford reminded her, "Now don't worry about that spot on your cheek."

Kathleen smiled warmly, "I won't, doctor, because *you* told me it was nothing to worry about."

This case illustrates the importance of the patient-physician relationship over time. Dr. Stafford had critical information about Kathleen, gained over a number of years. While Kathleen was adamant about not being a "bothersome patient," neither was she willing to just unconditionally accept his advice. She was intelligent and informed and wanted to take a role in her own care. He wove all this knowledge into his visit with her. He knew how close Kathleen and Al had been and how tenderly and stoically Kathleen had cared for Al. He also knew that Kathleen was more likely to take care of others than herself, and that she would only visit the office when absolutely necessary. He needed to make the most of the times when she came for prescription refills. He made sure that she knew that she was welcome at the office and that it was okay to talk about Al and her feelings of grief.

Kathleen felt comfortable enough to tell Dr. Stafford that she really didn't want to go to the Cancer Clinic. Had this not been the case, she might have chosen not to have the spot removed. Dr. Stafford's compassionate response reinforced for Kathleen that he took her concerns seriously. Kathleen's trust in Dr. Stafford is exemplified by her response at the end of the visit – "I am not going to worry because you told me not to."

40 Restoring the Healer

Sabrina Lim and Judith Belle Brown

Late one evening, Father Thomas, aged 68, came to the emergency room with signs and symptoms of a bowel obstruction. He had been playing golf when he experienced severe pain in his abdomen. He had also noticed that over the past month his bowel movements had not been very regular. He almost seemed embarrassed to tell me, a young female doctor, about his bowels. "It's a little embarrassing talking to you, you know, doctor," he said sheepishly. I smiled and said, "It doesn't bother me at all, but I could see how people might not be so comfortable talking about such private matters as their bowel movements." Father Thomas smiled warmly and softly chuckled. I decided to admit him to the hospital for routine treatment. At the time of his admission, I learned he was a retired priest.

His abdominal X-ray looked typical, and Father Thomas initially responded well to therapy. I saw him briefly every day to check his progress, and his history didn't suggest anything sinister. He wondered if his bowel difficulties were a result of change in his diet, as he no longer had a housekeeper to prepare nourishing meals for him since his retirement. "Since I have been cooking for myself, perhaps I have been a little extravagant," he admitted with a warm smile and soft chuckle. His only complaint beside the usual discomfort of having a tube up his nose was that he was hungry, since we had stopped feeding him to allow the bowel to rest and decompress. Father Thomas, a somewhat portly gentleman, told me, almost secretly, that he enjoyed his food. In response, I joked, "Even when I start to order food for you, you may not enjoy the hospital cuisine." Again the warm smile and soft chuckle served as his reply.

When Father Thomas failed to wean off his nasogastric tube, we went searching for another reason for his obstruction. During this time, Father Thomas was poked and prodded during a variety of investigations. His CT scan showed a metastatic colonic mass. He was not a candidate for surgery. Although we had extended diagnosing his cancer by only a week, I felt tremendous guilt that I had "missed it" when Father Thomas had been initially admitted to the hospital.

I had originally promised that he would be back on the golf course in a few short weeks. I learned during our daily visits that the game of golf had been a passion in his youth. But he had to forego this pleasure for many years as he devoted all his time to the demanding responsibilities of his large inner-city parish. Now, with his retirement unfolding before him, Father Thomas had renewed his love of the game. Sadly, there would be no more golf games. My guilt worsened as he seemed to quickly deteriorate following the diagnosis of inoperable cancer.

One early morning, after a particularly trying night on call, I stopped in with one of my medical students to see Father Thomas. As the student took the usual history, Father Thomas caught me staring out the sunny window of his room. Truthfully, I had never noticed the window in his room before. "What are you gazing at so intently, doctor?" he quietly inquired.

"Oh, I'm sorry Father," I quickly responded. I admitted to my inattention and told him that with all my long hours in the hospital, I had forgotten how beautiful the sun was.

With obvious effort Father Thomas readjusted his position in his hospital bed. Then, uncharacteristically, he pointedly asked, "But you're off call at noon, correct, doctor?"

"Yes, that's correct, I am off at noon, or at least once I get my rounds done," I replied.

In a more gentle tone, Father Thomas inquired, "And so doctor, what do you plan to do on this glorious, sun-filled day?"

I told him that although I was really tired from call, I wanted to enjoy this sunny day with my children. His warm smile and soft chuckle returned. "Then hurry up and go home, young lady! Enjoy the sun and play with your children." Father Thomas paused, and his face became serious. "Please savor the sun and the time with your children. Do it for me, if you will, as it is unlikely I will ever be able to enjoy such pleasures again," he said somberly. He appeared to know deep down it was very doubtful that he would ever leave the hospital. In that moment, I became overwhelmed by his generosity and felt that he had given me the forgiveness that I could not provide for myself.

I thanked him for his thoughtfulness. He in turn thanked me, and puzzled, I asked him why. "During the last few weeks in hospital," he explained, "I had forgotten what it felt like to be the one to heal another." Father Thomas paused momentarily, and then with reflection explained, "I have been in the role of a sick patient, not the role of priest, a role I have assumed for many, many years." Yet again his warm smile returned as he said, "Our talk today has restored me from the sick role to the role of healer." With conviction, Father Thomas concluded, "The ability to heal, to ameliorate another's suffering is something I cherish. So I thank you for helping me return to that place." He sunk back into his bed, appearing exhausted but content.

I could feel my eyes welling up with tears. I quickly patted his arm and told him that I would find time tomorrow at lunch to take him outside if he wished so he could enjoy the sunshine. Father Thomas quietly nodded and said that was fine, but for now I should enjoy the sun for him today.

He died the next day.

As I become more experienced in medicine, I often reflect on the early years of my career as a physician. I have learned as much about being a good physician from my patients as I have from my teachers and mentors. The patient-centered clinical method stresses the importance of understanding the whole person as well as the development of the patient-physician relationship. As I think about Father Thomas, he highlights for me the importance of recognizing the patient as a person first and how this relationship can heal not only the patient but the physician as well.

The Four Interactive Components of the Patient-Centered Clinical Method

Judith Belle Brown and Tanya Thornton

In the preceding four sections of this book, we focused on narratives that emphasized each separate component of the patient-centered clinical method. We recognize that the components cannot be portioned out, as the clinical method is an integrated and dynamic process. Therefore, the following stories in the final section of the book reflect the authors' attempts to explicate the complexity and synergy of the patient-centered clinical method by offering narratives that include two or more of the four interactive components of the method.

PREVIEW OF THE NARRATIVES

We begin with a story presented in two parts. Through the course of our careers, we witness much suffering and share in the losses experienced by our patients. In the midst of these tragedies, we often look for hope and seek to offer compassion. However, a patient's suicide is perhaps the most painful and potentially self-reflective experience we encounter in caring for our patients. This two-part story illuminates this experience.

The next narrative, **Chapter 43**, illustrates the therapeutic role inherent in the patient-doctor relationship, which can be healing when modern medicine fails to provide adequate treatment options. It also exemplifies the active role patients play in this healing process, when they are invited to equally participate in the treatment plan. Identification of roles and goals is essential to establishing common ground for the foundation of therapeutic success.

The following story, presented in two parts – **Chapter 44** and **Chapter 45** – is that of a healthy 18-year-old young woman. It is simple yet complex. The simplicity lies in the actual diagnosis and treatment – or so it seems. But as the story unravels, we observe how the four components of the patient-centered clinical method are not a seamless process but rather take this young woman down a rather bumpy road. In this journey from adolescence to adulthood she learns some valuable lessons about her health care needs. While her multiple health care providers may not have learned anything from their encounters with this feisty individual, we can be enlightened by her story.

In the next narrative, **Chapter 46**, the patient conceals her well-established diagnosis. Throughout the encounter with her new physician, she plants roadblocks. But why? The patient's story is a complex web of her battle with disease, her family's response to it, the challenges she endures and her physician's willingness to listen and learn. Together, patient and physician unlock doors – previously unimaginable.

How continuity of care bolsters the patient-physician relationship is underscored in **Chapter 47**. Continuity of care also provides a window into our patient's lives as we acquire more information and a deeper understanding of their context. How they respond to disease, the trajectory of their illness and their efforts to regain health become illuminated over time. Continuity, or knowing a person for an extended course of care, ultimately permits a greater appreciation of the whole person.

Time offers reflection, and often in the practice of family medicine, as well as other specialties caring for patients over an extended period, the unique opportunity of coming to know a person at a very intimate level provides remarkable insights. **Chapter 48** provides such an example. From the initial response of "oh no – my worst heartsink patient!" expressed during early encounters to the present "how good to see you," the many important aspects of being patient-centered are illuminated.

In the last two-part narrative, **Chapter 49** and **Chapter 50**, which comprise the final story in this book, we observe how the four interactive components of the patient-centered clinical method coalesce. We learn of this man's perceptions of his health, his vigilance over the control of his multiple diseases and finally his experience of illness. The patient's life experiences, as well as his proximal and distal contexts, play a dramatic role in his everyday health, the onset and perpetuation of his complex disease processes and his unique illness experience. While his traumatic past cannot be altered, his current contexts are amenable to change. Throughout the story, finding common ground is a constant challenge. Yet, as the physician learns more about her patient and comes to appreciate his disease and illness, as well as his aspirations for health, finding common ground becomes more attainable. Understanding the context in which he conducts his life also enhances the physician's ability to care for her patient from a patient-centered perspective. As the story reveals, the foundation of this evolving, complex and dynamic interchange is the patient-doctor relationship.

Narratives Illustrating the Four Interactive Components of the Patient-Centered Clinical Method

41 Looking for Hope – Finding Compassion: Part 1

Jane Uygur and Judith Belle Brown

I first met 73-year-old Derek when he was an inpatient on the geriatric psychiatry unit. I was the family physician who provided medical care for the psychiatric patients while they were hospitalized and was new to my role on the unit. The experienced nurses and psychiatrists were kindly guiding me in my care of their anxious and depressed elderly patients, and I was learning how to manage their multiple somatic complaints. There were many subtleties involved in distinguishing the need for reassurance versus the need to investigate. It was a challenging balance.

When Derek was readmitted to the unit, he learned very quickly that I was the new family doctor on staff. He found me at the nursing station and implored, "You're the new doctor! I have this terrible pain. I need your help. Please, can you do something for me?" Derek was redirected by one of the nurses to return to his room and reassured that I would come to see him shortly.

The head nurse, Mary, turned to me and stated in a matter-of-fact tone, "That's Derek. He has been in here many times. We know him very well. He's depressed and anxious and very somatic. He often complains of abdominal pain." As I rose to commence my rounds, I decided to go and see Derek first. After all, his anxiety was contagious.

When I entered his dark room, Derek was lying on the bed. In a strained voice, his litany of complaints began, "Doctor, I have these terrible cramps. I'm so constipated. I can't go to the washroom. And I'm having such a hard time going pee. It doesn't seem to matter how much water I drink, I can't pee. Please help me. All the nurses do is give me Tylenol and tell me to lie down."

I conducted a systematic review of his complaints. Nothing added up. Derek felt like a collection of riddles that I could not unravel. He was constipated, but he had had a BM just yesterday. He couldn't pee, but sometimes he was peeing too much. The abdominal pain didn't fit any pattern. I was unable to come up with an easy answer. He was obviously quite somatically preoccupied. I wondered if I should do a few tests just to make sure I wasn't missing anything and maybe reassure him too. I offered, "Maybe we should do a few tests just to check things out."

Derek quickly retorted, "I've had lots of tests. I just want something for the pain."

Then Derek went through the long list of treatments that hadn't worked. There didn't seem to be much left that we could do. "Well, let me think about what I can do for you, Derek. I'll see you again later this week," I stated as I headed for the door.

"But I need something for the pain, now!" cried Derek.

All I could say was, "Let me see what I can do." It was a struggle to extract myself from the room.

After seeing my other patients, I returned to the nursing station. Derek was there again. "Please, doctor, give me something for the pain," he begged. Derek was redirected by one of the nurses, and I tried to shrink down out of view.

As I started to write a few orders for Derek, Mary, the head nurse, peered over my shoulder and said, "He's had an abdominal ultrasound last admission, you know. His urine test was clear last week."

"Oh," I said.

"We're trying not to reward his behavior with attention. He needs to be redirected," Mary concluded, walking away. So I thought to myself, "*What am I supposed to do?*" I felt a little helpless.

Then his psychiatrist came on the ward. "Hey Mark," I said, "I met Derek today."

"Mmm," said Mark. Mark knew Derek very well over the course of his many admissions and provided some background. Derek had suffered intractable depression for over four years. He had overdosed several times. He had been tried on numerous psychotropic medications and even ECT. Small gains were made, but Derek's depression never fully went into remission.

Derek's past history revealed that he had been brought up in a home with an unavailable father and a somatically preoccupied and anxious mother. Despite this, he experienced many successes as an athlete and later as a lawyer. However, relationships had always been a challenge. Derek had been married three times. His first wife, with whom he had three children, had divorced him. His second wife had died of cancer. He then met his third and current wife, Joan. She continued to stand by him, but the relationship was strained.

I asked Mark, "So all his somatic complaints have been investigated?"

With a heavy sigh, Mark replied, "Oh yes, he's had loads of tests and done the rounds with the specialists. Everything has come back looking fine."

There really didn't seem to be much that I could do. Twice a week I did rounds on the unit, and each time, Derek was waiting for me. If I didn't visit him first he would follow me into another patient's room with his complaints. If I did see him first, he would seek me out again and again at the nursing station with the same litany of complaints and pleas for help. Other patients would also seek me out and have numerous somatic complaints. However, for them, there were things to investigate, symptomatic treatments to try, reassurance to give and hope that their depression would improve. There wasn't any of that for Derek.

And at times I would reach my limit of patience. I felt angry, and as my sense of impotence escalated, I thought, "*He's sucking me dry! It's all about him! Leave me alone!*" There were days when it was all I could do to muster a civil attempt at reassurance and depart. I had tried to help Derek to understand that his physical pain was a reflection of his emotional pain. But it didn't work.

Then Derek was discharged. His wife couldn't cope with him at home, but he was too stable to remain in the hospital. Arrangements were made for him to go into a nursing home. I felt a huge sense of relief, but a pang of remorse remained.

A few weeks later, Derek was readmitted to the hospital. He had walked out of the nursing home into the middle of a busy street, stating he wanted to kill himself. No harm had come to him, but the nursing home refused to take him back. Derek's suicide attempt jarred me out of my frustration with him. He had obviously been in a great deal of emotional pain to contemplate suicide. My empathy returned.

When I asked Derek if he would try again, he said firmly, "I'd never try to throw myself in front of a car again. I'd feel too bad for the person that hit me. What if they got injured? How would they feel knowing they had killed someone?" It was comforting to hear that Derek could think about someone other than himself. For the first time I wondered what Derek had been like before he'd become ill.

So I made it my objective to discover if I could find more glimpses of the Derek that was buried under the depression. It was very hard to get him to talk about anything other than his bodily functions. Every now and then I'd find a clue in his conversation. Sometimes if I enquired further he would expand.

"These cramps are killing me. Is there anything you can do? Look at this belly. I'm gaining too much weight. I think it is the medication they have me on. I used to be so fit," Derek rambled.

"How did you used to keep fit?" I asked tentatively, hoping this might be a fruitful avenue to learn more about Derek's strengths.

"Tennis," Derek answered flatly. "I used to play a lot."

And then the litany of complaints would begin again. Slowly though, I started to get an image of who Derek was, who he had been. But I was still frustrated. There was little I could do, but seeing Derek as a person rather than a patient made it easier to empathize and care for him.

Derek underwent another round of ECT. He was a little less anxious and agitated but still somatically preoccupied. His suicidal ideation stabilized. Then I got the news. He was being transferred to another nursing home, the one I worked at. He was going to be on my floor. He was going to be under my care, my patient – indefinitely. He was only 73, young for a nursing home. He was in relatively good physical health. He could be there for a long time. I have to admit I was trying not to despair.

Jane Uygur and Judith Belle Brown

It was hard for Derek to settle into the nursing home. He didn't want to be there. He wanted to be at home with his wife, Joan. "Everyone is so much older than I am," Derek would moan, "and I have no one to talk to." Once again, Derek started expressing some suicidal ideation but admitted that he couldn't go through with it. However, the staff was concerned about his suicide risk, and it was decided that Derek should wear a wander guard to alert us if he was going off of the floor. Although humiliated, Derek was clever enough to find scissors and cut the wander guard off. We put it on again and hid the scissors elsewhere. I felt conflicted. While the wander guard served to protect Derek's life, it was also a profound humiliation. He was like a caged animal.

While the nursing home staff was undeniably worried about Derek's suicidal ideation, they were also very frustrated by the constant somatization and his repeated requests for p.r.n. medication. At our weekly rounds, Derek was always at the top of the list. But we became more adept in ascertaining what was passive versus active suicidal ideation. While Derek's anxiety remained constant, at least the staff's worries waned.

During the first few months of Derek's stay in the nursing home I felt like I was constantly "putting out fires." I spent a lot of time reassuring staff, trying to educate them, trying to establish some sense of trust between Derek, me and the rest of the team. It was exhausting.

Then things seemed to settle for a while. Derek continued to have the same complaints. I saw him every week. Again, my feeling of hopelessness returned. What could I do for this man? I had nothing to offer him. I couldn't even reassure him. No matter how often I told him that his pain was not indicative of any fatal illness, he was never free from worry.

I decided to meet Derek weekly, for approximately 20–30 minutes. During these visits I was committed to letting Derek know that I could see that he was suffering and that I knew his suffering was real. I would try to understand what his illness meant to him and explore what was driving his pain. I was determined to be fully present and mindful during our sessions. And to give him hope.

I just wasn't sure how to give Derek hope. After all, it was a hopeless case. Twenty percent of people with depression do not respond to treatment, and Derek seemed to be one of them. How can you provide hope when you feel hopeless? After a lot of thought, I decided to provide Derek with hope by letting him know during our weekly visits that I hadn't given up on him. I would continue to find ways to make him feel better. To convince him of this I would occasionally order a test to reassure him, or try a different medication to relieve one of his symptoms.

And so the next few months passed. Our weekly visits would go something like this:

Derek would begin, "I've got cramps."

"Are they like your usual cramps?" I would ask.

"Yes." He would flatly answer.

"Are you worried about them?" I would gently inquire.

"Yes." His response was more pointed.

Reassuringly I would suggest, "You've had them for a long time, and they usually settle in a few days. You have always had relief from them for a time."

"But I can't stand the pain. I'm afraid it could be cancer," Derek would say, the fear mounting in his voice.

"I don't think it is cancer," I would calmly reply. "The tests you have had have never shown any signs of cancer."

"It's been a long time since I had a test," Derek would state indignantly.

"Well, it is over six months since we did an ultrasound. To reassure you, I can repeat the ultrasound," I would offer.

"Okay. But what about the pain?" was Derek's mournful reply.

Our visits continued in this vein. On some days he was more somatic than others, but in general he was able to engage in more "normal" conversation. I enjoyed the visits when he was open to discussing his past life. However, he was still hopeless about his future and distraught about spending his life in the nursing home. During some of our visits he was content with exchanging just a few words. He didn't always want to talk for a long time.

The last time I saw him he was quite distressed about having a bout of diarrhea. I tried to reassure him that it would pass. I told him we would "hold" his laxatives. He then began to worry that he would get constipated. We talked it through and at the end of the session I said, as I always did, "I haven't given up on you. I'm still working to make you feel better. I'll see you next Thursday, Derek."

And he answered back, as he often did, "I don't know if I'll make it until then."

The day before my next Thursday visit, in the middle of my busy clinic, I was called to the phone. It was the medical director of the nursing home.

"Derek died last night. There are some unanswered questions about the death. It appears he may have jumped. Did you have any suspicion he was suicidal?" the director asked over the phone.

Shocked by this news, I stammered, "Umm, ah, well, no. I mean he had an intractable depression, but he hadn't been actively suicidal lately." My mind raced through recent events, evaluating whether they might provide some clues, but I could see none.

"Well, if you think of anything that might shed some light on the issue, could you let me know? We're going to have to investigate this," concluded the director as he signed off.

And then I cried. I cried because Derek was gone. Derek, who I had seen almost every week for two years. Derek, who I genuinely liked and cared about. Then came the wave of nausea. This was my first suicide. *"Did I miss something?" "Will they find me at fault?" "Will the family want to sue me?"* And then I felt selfish that I should even be worrying about myself.

I finished up at the clinic and went to the nursing home. I read the note from the physician who had called the code blue when Derek jumped. It hadn't initially been clear that he had jumped. Some witnesses had said they could have sworn that he just fell over the railing. The injuries were too extensive for that. He was bleeding from the nose and head. He appeared to have fractured both of his legs. Derek was still conscious when the doctor arrived at his side. His last words were "I jumped." He was taken away by ambulance and died from his injuries en route to the hospital.

Then I visualized the whole series of events – the planning, the jump, the injuries, Derek's last words. I visualized it over and over again. How brutal. How violent. For Derek, who always said he was a coward, how much emotional pain had he been suffering to do that to himself? How ugly, relentless, and inescapable that pain must have been. I felt I had never really understood how horrific Derek's pain had been for him.

He must have given us signs and we had missed them. I scoured the chart. No, Derek was always depressed, sometimes passively suicidal, but there had been no clues that his ideation was escalating. Maybe he had gotten well enough to take the initiative to jump? Maybe he was just tired of it all and he was clever enough to know how to end it without giving himself away? I would never know.

He had been a tortured soul.

As the days passed, I started thinking about my role as healer in Derek's case. I couldn't help thinking about my "treatment plan of hope." What a crock! Who was I trying to fool? Derek knew it was hopeless. I knew it was hopeless. What good was it? Had I deluded myself that offering false hope was an act of healing?

But maybe it wasn't wrong to look for hope in a hopeless situation. Maybe it wasn't about hope at all. Maybe it was really just about caring for Derek and finding compassion. I was learning to be a healer, a good healer. Maybe I was learning that some wounds are just too deep. I was learning the art of compassion.

43 Itching to Be Treated

Tanya Thornton

"Rosa?" I called out into the crowded waiting room. I checked my daysheet: Rosa Medeiros – itchy rash. I looked up. From the corner of the room, my eye caught some movement: a slight woman, mid-20s, well-kept. She stood up and started gathering her belongings: coat, boots, purse and briefcase. Avoiding eye contact, she glanced my way and hurried over.

"I'm Dr. Griffiths, pleased to meet you," I said, guiding her into the exam room. She took a seat without speaking, dropping her mass of belongings to the floor, a stray curl popping out of her well-manicured ponytail.

"What brings you in today?"

Without smiling, her small voice replied, "I need help."

"Sure. What can I do for you today?" I asked, realizing that this wasn't as straightforward as the itchy rash my daysheet had alluded to.

"I need help to stop picking my arms," she answered, looking up sheepishly.

"Tell me more about your arms."

"I feel horrible with myself, frustrated. I wish I could stop, I *need* to stop." She started to sob and heaved a breath. "I know it makes scars … it's like a storm cloud overhead, I can't break free, and I have only until June."

"Why June?"

"I'm getting married June 15th," she replied, slowing her breathing. "I want to look beautiful; I don't want Mark to see these ugly arms and change his mind."

"Tell me about Mark," I probed. This line of questioning brought comfort, and she looked directly into my eyes as she described her fiancé and pending wedding. At 29, she thought she'd never find the "right guy," then one day at the local coffee shop, they connected and "the rest is history," she finished.

"Five years later, and I'm planning the dream of my life. I should be happy. Don't get me wrong, I am, but every time I get excited, I get scared. My heart races, I start to breathe fast, and sometimes I can't catch my breath. I wonder what people will whisper at my wedding about my scars. My arms are so ugly." The tears started again. I passed the tissue box.

Glancing at the clock, I realized the quick start to my day, the "itchy rash" booked for 15 minutes, was going to put me behind. Then, my own thoughts of staying on time and efficiency were interrupted with Rosa's plea, "So, can you help me? Is there enough time before June?"

What am I doing worrying about the clock, I chastised myself. "Do you think there is a medicine that could help?" Rosa asked. Then she noticed that I wasn't paying attention. "I could come back if you're busy," she said quietly.

"Oh no, I was just thinking," I replied, embarrassed. "Yes, there are treatments, but tell me more," I reassured, not really knowing what the treatments were, but convincing myself that she couldn't possibly be the first patient with this condition.

Rosa eagerly continued on, "It's like an addiction. When the urge comes, I just can't stop. I pick, usually when I'm on the couch watching TV. I feel awful afterwards. Yesterday, I was rude at work. Last night was the worst: I sat there picking for a whole hour! It's like I have to take it out on myself for being mean with my co-workers. When my arm started to bleed, I felt disgusted with myself. I wish I could feel better. I feel lousy all the time." The tears started again.

"Do you ever feel so lousy that you might want to end your life?" I asked tentatively.

"Oh no, I'm not crazy, at least not like my sister – I just want to feel better."

Her sister. Hmm. Family history of psychiatric problems. I made a mental note to explore this further. *Should I do that today? What time is it?* I casted a furtive glance at the clock – I succeeded, she was looking down. *Only five minutes overtime so far, okay, better explore the mental health history now,* I decided.

Rosa recounted her childhood: single mom, older sister, both seeing doctors for treatment of manic depression. Despite suffering from symptoms of anxiety and irritability at times, she did not fulfill the criteria for any psychiatric disorder and instead, was allocated into a diagnostic black hole – episodic symptoms without classification. Rosa believed she was "the healthy one," taking care of household responsibilities when her mom and sister "got sick." She gained a sense of accomplishment in this role. *Rosa* was the survivor, the resilient one in times of family crisis. She viewed her pending marriage as a source of reassurance that she *was* normal. She distinguished this from her mother's life, which was without support. This sense of independence and a unique identity from that of her family had, in the past, provided her with optimism during thoughts of self-doubt and skin picking.

"It scares me now to think I might be losing control of my life. I've worked hard to get here. I want to be happy. I have a great job, a fantastically supportive fiancé – what's wrong with me? What if I lose this all, just because I can't control my picking? What if Mark stops loving me once he knows the real me?" she implored.

"If he loves you, he will stick by you," I superficially replied, now realizing that I was even further behind schedule. I was frustrated that I hadn't yet helped her, and time was running out. *Do I have time to look up treatments for skin picking in my office library? Definitely not right now,* I realized. *Will she come back if I don't have an answer for her today? It was worth the risk asking,* I decided.

"Rosa, I think we have enough time between now and June to deal with your skin picking," I said, trying to exude more confidence in my plan than I was feeling. "What do you think about coming back next week to talk about this some more? In the meantime, I'll look into what the latest treatments are, and which ones might be best for you. I'd really like to chat again and hear about your wedding plans."

"I'd like that," Rosa replied, cracking a smile for the first time in 30 minutes. *We connected. What had I said that made her trust me? I didn't offer a specific solution for her problem, or send her home with any medication that she could try in the next week. In essence, I felt I had gathered information and offered nothing in return for her story.*

She came to my office with a candid plea for help. It was clear that she expected me to have a solution for her skin-picking problem, and it was obvious during the exchange that there wasn't a specific therapy offered by myself at the end of the visit. And yet, she was smiling at the end, shaking my hand, thanking me. *What happened in those 30 minutes to make her think I had helped her?*

As I reflected on that visit, I realized it was *the connection, the relationship* that enabled Rosa to return for follow-up visits. She felt I *heard* her fears, *understood* her anxieties or simply cared.

In subsequent visits, we learned *together* that much of the treatment revolved around support systems, stress management and cognitive behavioral counseling. Although there was one case report of antidepressant medications being helpful, emphasis was placed on treatments such as understanding her illness through education, habit reversal training and social connections. I looked at this list of therapies and realized that each one was facilitated through the patient-family physician relationship, *not* by a quick-fix pill.

A desire for self-control is a feature of most illnesses. It is why one of the fundamental beliefs that physicians have traditionally guarded is the maintenance of personal autonomy during therapy for an illness. In our initial encounter, her concerns were validated. During subsequent visits, Rosa played a central role in choosing therapies. Her ideas, goals and roles were respected and supported. Perhaps *this* is why she found our visits therapeutic, despite modest success in the treatment of her skin picking disorder.

Rosa and Mark were married on June 15th, as planned. She looked stunning in her long-sleeved gown with fingertip lace. Mark continues to stick by Rosa – the woman he loves.

44 Not a Typical Teenager – Part 1

Bridget L. Ryan

Gwen was an intelligent, articulate, healthy 18-year-old young woman with just two weeks and three exams ahead of her before she graduated from high school. While walking to the park on a Monday afternoon in late June to meet a friend, she experienced a sharp pain in her left shoulder. By the time she reached the park, she knew that something was not right. She exclaimed to her friend, "This pain is brutal."

Gwen called her mother, Joyce, on her cell phone. Joyce suggested that Gwen should go to the emergency room of their local hospital. "Call Dr. Young's office. You'll likely get the after-hours service. You can check with the nurse to see if they think going to the ER is the best thing to do. I'll meet you at the hospital." The on-call nurse agreed that Gwen should go directly to the ER. And so began Gwen's journey through the health care system.

When Gwen arrived at the ER, she was seen by the triage nurse who asked her level of pain. "It is a 10. The pain is in my left shoulder and it is making it hard for me to breathe." The nurse asked if Gwen had any idea what might be wrong. Gwen replied, "I don't know. I have scoliosis, but this isn't like any pain I've had before."

Gwen waited in the ER for three anxious hours until she was seen by a physician. When he asked her level of pain, Gwen replied, "It is a four now."

The doctor examined her back carefully. He checked her reflexes. "I think it is likely just a muscle spasm."

When the doctor left the examining room, Gwen told her mother she was worried. "I don't feel comfortable leaving. It doesn't feel like a muscle spasm."

When the doctor returned, her mother insisted, "Can you check further? My daughter isn't feeling comfortable about leaving." The doctor reluctantly agreed to order blood work.

After waiting another two hours with no evidence of any further action regarding the blood work, Gwen said to her mom, "I want to go. I'm tired, and I'm just done in." They returned home, where Gwen went to bed and slept until late the next day.

Gwen returned to school Wednesday and found herself once again short of breath and exhausted. She made an appointment with her family physician for the next day. The family physician listened to her story and suggested that it might be a collapsed lung. He initially ordered a chest X-ray, but then decided that the collapsed lung was unlikely: "Given your overall health and your age, I think it likely is just a muscle spasm," he said. Instead, the doctor ordered an X-ray of her back as a routine follow-up of her scoliosis. Having been told twice by two different physicians that her problem was a muscle spasm, Gwen assumed that it must indeed be a muscle spasm.

Gwen returned to school again on Friday but by mid-morning could not tolerate the pain. She called her family physician and asked if she could get the chest X-ray after all. Her family physician agreed, and Gwen went for the X-ray.

When Gwen returned home later that day, there was a message on the answering machine from her family physician stating that she had a 10% collapsed lung. The voice message went on to explain, "This shouldn't be causing much shortness of breath and should heal on its own. However, you should rest. If it doesn't get better or it gets worse, you should go to the ER."

But Gwen was unsure how to know if it was worse or not better. "*How long should I wait?*" she wondered. "*It's already been a week, so maybe it will be better soon. I think I will just wait until Monday and see how it goes.*" Gwen spent the weekend in bed.

By Monday she was no better and after once again attempting to go to school, she left early and went with her mother to the ER. Arriving at 10:00 a.m., this time Gwen told the triage nurse that she had a 10% collapsed lung and was seen sooner than on her last visit. An X-ray and some blood work were ordered; however, Gwen was informed that she would have to go to the other local hospital because this specialty service was not offered at their hospital: "You might need a chest tube – the thoracic surgeon at the other hospital can throw one in, and you can go home tonight." Gwen was given an envelope containing her chest X-ray and blood work results and was driven by her mother to the other hospital at 3:00 p.m.

Throughout her two visits to the ER, Gwen had felt dismissed by the staff. She wondered if they viewed her as just an overreacting teenager. No one asked her about her breathing after she mentioned it to the triage nurse. Gwen later questioned if she herself was to blame for being given the wrong diagnosis: "*Maybe I got it backwards, I should have said that my breathing was bad and that this was causing my shoulder pain.*" She also wondered if they took her concerns less seriously because she said her pain had decreased to a four. Ironically, because she had a collapsed lung, her pain decreased because she had been sitting in the waiting room for three hours. Her pain increased with exertion.

At this point, no one had asked Gwen what effect the pain was having on her life. She had made repeated attempts to go to school and "tough it out." She had accepted that it was just a muscle spasm and there was nothing that could be done but to take anti-inflammatories and rest. She was in her second-last week of high school and was very stressed about her final exams. Despite desperately wanting to, she was unable to attend school. Understanding her context would have been an indication of how much distress she was experiencing. At this point, it had been eight days since the onset of her pain. A more patient-centered approach – one that attended to the illness experience and Gwen as a whole person – might have led to a more prompt and accurate diagnosis.

Now having a definitive diagnosis, Gwen entered the treatment phase of her journey through the health care system.

45 Not a Typical Teenager – Part 2

Bridget L. Ryan

Eighteen-year-old Gwen drove with her mother to meet with the thoracic surgeon at the other local hospital. They sat in the ER waiting room for another anxious and uncertain four hours until Gwen was seen by the thoracic surgeon at 8:00 p.m. After some curt introductions and a review of her presenting problem, the surgeon stated, "Normally, a collapsed lung will heal itself within 72 hours. So you can choose to wait a bit longer or have the chest tube inserted tonight."

Gwen was unsure what to do – she had been in debilitating pain for eight days and was feeling very stressed about the amount of school she had already missed. Perhaps having the chest tube inserted now would be the answer. She thought to herself, "*I'll get this done, be home by tonight and get back to school tomorrow.*"

The chest tube was successfully inserted under a local anesthetic. However, Gwen was shocked when the surgeon informed her that she would have to spend the night in hospital for monitoring. On the other hand, she was exhausted and groggy after the procedure and actually relieved when she was finally admitted to the thoracic ward at midnight.

Gwen did not sleep well through the night, but the next morning, the day nurse was very helpful and Gwen began to rally a bit. The nurse realized that Gwen was an independent teenager who wanted to be well and took her for a brief walk to test her strength. She also told Gwen, "If you want, you can talk to a social worker. They can be really helpful when it comes to things like getting your school stuff organized. She can even give you a note to take back to your school." Unfortunately, once the nurse went off duty, no one else raised this referral option with Gwen, and she did not feel comfortable in asking to see the social worker.

Gwen spent another night in the hospital to ensure an optimal recovery from the procedure. Upon discharge, she was given Tylenol with codeine for pain and told that she could return to school the next day. No one explained what to expect with respect to the normal healing process, what to be concerned about, or any possible side effects from the medication.

Being very independent and wanting to exercise some control over her situation, Gwen insisted on doing as much as possible for herself. As a result, on a number of occasions while in the hospital, she was told that she was "such an easy patient." The difficulty was that everyone assumed that the easy patient didn't have any real needs because she was not complaining. Unfortunately, no one at the hospital had attended to Gwen's school concerns stemming from her illness. The day nurse had suggested a referral to the social worker, but there was no follow-up.

Also, Gwen was given very little information about what to do or what to expect when she went home. No one warned her that she might feel groggy and nauseous from the medication. No one told her that she might continue to be tired for a while. Instead, she was led to believe that she would rebound the next day and return to school. Contrary to what she had been told, she was not able to attend school until the following week. She stopped taking the Tylenol #3 after only one day because of the nausea and because her pain control was not ideal. Gwen's needs concerning her after-care were not met.

When Gwen returned to school the following week, she discovered that she was expected to write her examinations despite her two-week absence and her ongoing fatigue. Her stress level, already very high, rapidly increased. In a panic, she called her family physician and was able to get an appointment that afternoon. She explained to her doctor, "I just can't write the exams. I've missed two weeks of classes, and I still need to nap every day."

Her doctor readily agreed, "You're not strong enough physically or mentally to write your exams now." He provided her with a note outlining her condition and her limitations. Her school agreed that her examination period would be extended. Gwen could finally concentrate on taking care of herself and healing from both her illness and her experience of the health care system.

Gwen learned that she needed to be an advocate for herself throughout this illness journey. She had been labeled an "easy patient" and as such was often "overlooked." However, on two occasions she took matters into her own hands: first, Gwen called her family physician and requested the chest X-ray, which became the key to her diagnosis. Fortunately, her family physician was responsive to her request. Gwen advocated for herself a second time when she sought out her family physician's help because she was not well enough to write her exams. She gained valuable experience in navigating the health care system. Along the way, Gwen met some helpful and competent providers, but her care was chaotic and disconnected, and her context was ignored. This led to delays and miscommunication, both of which added to the burden of her illness experience.

Gwen's story illustrates the four components of the patient-centered clinical method. With respect to exploring Gwen's perceptions of her health, as well as her disease and illness experience, Gwen did not receive an accurate or timely diagnosis of her symptoms. Though she interacted with a number of providers, no one asked about her illness experience. No one explored her feelings, her ideas, the effect of the collapsed lung on her functioning, or her expectations. In fact, her idea that this was not typical scoliosis pain was ignored.

In terms of understanding the whole person, Gwen's context was neither explored nor understood. She was approaching high school final examinations and determined to return to school as soon as possible. An exploration of her context could have led to a better understanding of the degree of disability caused by the pain she experienced. From Gwen's perspective, she was viewed as a "typical teenage girl" prone to exaggeration, hence her complaint was minimized when she first presented to the ER. It is important when caring for adolescents to remember that, although they may share developmental similarities, they are all unique individuals.

Health care providers need to recognize that adolescents, like many adult patients, may not always know how best to articulate their needs. Thus, some exploration of their illness experience and context will ensure that their needs are met. This case illustrates the complex context in which adolescents live and experience illness. Some of this context exists outside the realm of the health care system, but some of it can be caused *by* the health care system.

A lack of finding common ground around treatment and management is all too well illustrated by this case. There was no initial common ground with respect to diagnosis, and indeed there was a significant delay in receiving the correct diagnosis – and during this time Gwen became convinced, against her better judgment, that she had only a muscle spasm. Once diagnosed and treated, there was little in the way of finding common ground. She was told at one hospital that the insertion of a chest tube was an outpatient procedure, and then without any regard for the impact on Gwen, she was told at the other hospital that she would need to be admitted. There was minimal discussion around what Gwen could expect upon discharge. She was given conflicting messages regarding how much school she could anticipate missing and what sort of healing process she might expect.

The patient-physician relationship is illustrated both positively and negatively in this case. Unfortunately, Gwen's family physician did not immediately order the chest X-ray. Once her condition was diagnosed, the communication of the diagnosis and what she should do through a voice message on Friday evening was not ideal. However, on the two occasions when Gwen called upon her family physician to advocate on her behalf, he responded appropriately and compassionately.

Adolescence is a time of change and growth. It is also a time when adolescents begin to take responsibility for their own health care needs. A patient-centered approach is important, because adolescents require health care providers who consider them as unique persons with their own context and needs. Adolescents also require health care providers who are willing to explain and discuss diagnoses and treatments with them so that their care is coordinated and understood.

46 More Than Just a Tummy Ache

Lemmese Al-Watban and Judith Belle Brown

It was approaching the end of the day, and I had one more patient on my list to see: "Asha … stomach pain." As I looked through her chart, I found no previous medical history. Her last appointment was two years ago, and her medication list only mentioned oral contraception. I breathed in a deep sigh of relief. She would probably be a simple case of the stomach flu. I was finally starting to feel relaxed. I had been so anxious all day, as this was my first day in practice after completing residency. Little did I know that I was going to meet one of my most challenging patients.

Thirty-year-old Asha presented to the clinic because she had been experiencing stomach pain for two weeks. She described how the pain was not constant and how she felt bloated and constipated. She denied any previous medical issues and felt that nothing had recently changed in her life. There seemed to be no alarming symptoms, and she appeared to be in good health. She had looked up her symptoms on the Internet and was convinced that she had parasites! As we continued to talk, I could not help but notice that she was not moving her left arm.

"Is there something wrong with your arm, Asha?" I inquired.

"Oh … it's paralyzed. I have MS … but it has been in remission for a while. My stomach pain has nothing to do with it!" she replied in a matter-of-fact tone.

Asha went on to tell me how excited she was about her upcoming appointment with Dr. Yong, her neurologist. She was going to have Botox injected into her paralyzed arm to relieve the pain. Asha had delayed this decision for over two years because she wanted to get pregnant. Now that her baby girl, Jana, was a year old, she felt the time was right to try the Botox. I found her initial concealment of her multiple sclerosis (MS) unusual, but did not think much of it at the time. We ended that visit with her demanding to be tested for parasites. Although I was not convinced of that diagnosis, I felt pressured into ordering the lab tests.

At the end of the week, Asha's tests came back negative for parasites. She was relieved to hear this news and seemed to agree with me that her symptoms were probably related to a mild case of constipation. She was willing to try a short course of laxatives and agreed to follow up with me in a week.

The next morning, Asha surprised me with a visit to the clinic, appearing anxious and tearful.

"The laxative didn't work, doctor!" Before I could explain to her that laxatives take some time to work, she yelled, "I can't take this anymore! I have a baby to take care of at home!" As she started to cry, Asha muttered, "I think I might have ovarian cancer." We sat down and I began to explore if there was any reason for her to think that she might have cancer. I wondered if there was something going on in her life that was provoking her anxiety and contributing to her abdominal pain. *Was she depressed? Were things okay at home?*

Each time I endeavored to inquire about her personal life or her mood, Asha avoided answering and insisted I concentrate on her complaint. She had looked up her symptoms once again on the Internet and was certain: if she did not have parasites, then she surely had ovarian cancer. Although Asha had no family history of cancer and her symptoms were too short-lived to jump to that diagnosis, I feared that my lack of clinical experience might result in missing such a fatal diagnosis. As it is known that ovarian cancer is notorious for being difficult to diagnose, I saw no harm in fulfilling her request for a pelvic ultrasound. Better safe than sorry.

Over the next few weeks I was absent from the clinic. To my astonishment, when I returned there was a pile of reports on my desk concerning Asha. She had been to the emergency room a couple times with abdominal pain. Two pelvic ultrasounds were performed, demonstrating a small right ovarian cyst. I had received one letter from Dr. Kim and another from Dr. Tran, both gynecologists she had seen in the same week regarding the cyst. They had both reassured her that the cyst was benign and advised no further management.

Seeing Asha's lengthy paper trail made me even more convinced that there was something else going on. I was expecting to see her that very afternoon for her follow-up appointment and was preparing myself to confront her with my concerns about psychological or social causes for her symptoms. But Asha never appeared. When I called her at home, she informed me how much better she was feeling since she started seeing a herbalist. The herbalist had diagnosed parasites and put her on a bowel cleanse. I let her know that although her herbalist was treating her now, I would still like to be involved in her care and if she felt the need to talk, I would listen.

I felt defeated and frustrated. Both the herbalist and I prescribed the same solution for her problem (laxatives), but Asha preferred the herbalist's assessment and treatment.

Many thoughts went through my head: *Did I fail my patient? Was I less of a healer than the herbalist? Was I wrong to think that psychosocial issues could be the cause? Was it truly a missed case of parasites?* Part of me felt that more was under the surface; it wasn't just a parasite infection. *But what was it?* I had so many unanswered questions: *Why did she hide her MS at the beginning? Was she afraid her new symptoms were part of the MS and she was in denial? Was she merely worried about her Botox treatment failing?*

Although I did not see Asha for some time, I continued to receive letters from her neurologist, updating me on her progress. The Botox was initially successful and her pain had improved, but unfortunately, it did not last long.

Several months passed before Asha returned to the clinic. This time, something was different about her: she had lost her tenacity and her spirit seemed crushed. "Doctor, do you remember when you told me I could talk to you?"

"Yes, what is wrong?"

This time Asha spoke, and I listened.

Asha had been diagnosed with MS three years ago. It all started a week after her marriage to Eric. She was rushed to the emergency room with what was initially thought to be a right-sided stroke. A couple days into her hospital admission, she was given the bad news. "Asha, you have MS." With those few words, her entire life turned upside down. Eric was devastated. He was unable to handle what this meant and feared he would not be capable of caring for Asha. They separated for a while. In an effort to save her marriage and keep the man she loved, Asha assured her husband that she would not allow this disease to change her life. Since Eric wanted to have children, she delayed her Botox treatments until after she got pregnant. Asha endured her pain in silence and constantly put on a brave face. After her daughter, Jana, was born, Asha found it increasingly difficult to manage. In desperation, Asha asked her mother to move in with them in order to help her care for her young infant. But Eric was angry about Asha's mother living with them and constantly threatened to leave.

Asha had invested so much hope in her expectation that the Botox would relieve her pain. Having pain relief would allow her to manage on her own again and regain some normalcy in her turmoil-ridden marriage. The idea that the Botox treatment might not work had terrified her to the degree that it made her feel ill. Although the Botox treatment was successful for a couple of months, the pain soon returned, this time even stronger, but Eric's lack of support and avoidance hurt Asha even more. Then Asha discovered Eric was having an affair. There was no hope for reconciliation.

Although she was now going through the trauma of divorce proceedings, Asha felt as if a burden had been lifted off her shoulders. "No longer do I need to hide behind a mask; I can be myself," said Asha confidently.

Often in the practice of medicine we meet people who are ill and suffering without a clear disease. Despite our efforts to understand their illness experiences, we are faced with locked doors, either because we have not found the right keys or because the patient was not ready to let us in. Whatever the case, gaining the patient's trust is the first step in creating a healing patient-doctor relationship.

The ability to have patience is also important. Patients need their own time to heal, and as doctors we need to appreciate each individual's readiness and be patient with them yet persistent in trying to understand their suffering. We hold a key that with a little bit of practice can open most doors. Only by attentive listening to our patients' narratives and genuine caring for their suffering are we able to understand the meaning of their illnesses.

47 Continuity Equals Care

Adrienne Watson and Judith Belle Brown

Another new patient. One in a stream of many, as I had just opened my practice. I called him from the waiting room, introduced myself on the way down the hall, and then our journey began.

As a relatively new graduate in family medicine when I first met Arun, I remember being intimidated by the number of medical problems he presented with. Just in his late-30s, he had already had rhabdomyolysis and been in a coma, which was complicated by a myocardial infarction. He had a multitude of other complex medical problems. I remember thinking, *"How on earth am I ever going to be able to manage his numerous medical problems?"*

I tried to hide my nervousness and discomfort, but as he spoke, I became increasingly anxious. Rhabdo in a 30-something year old? Previous myocardial infarction? Seizures? Cervical disc herniation with chronic pain and Raynaud's? Hyperlipidemia, hypertension and depression? Multiple drug sensitivities? Yet somehow he looked healthy and quite happy. Where was I to begin? The prospect was daunting. Medical school had not prepared me for this. Yet something made me rise to this challenge rather than cowering in fear, as I was certainly tempted to do. Arun was there, asking for my help. He had seen so many doctors in the past, and it was my chance to try and help him along. I was not at all ready for it. But, here he was. My most complicated young patient to date.

So we began. When we embarked on the process of addressing his numerous illnesses, it seemed as though there were so many roadblocks. The internist didn't listen to him and made him decidedly uncomfortable, to the point where he was in tears and refused to go back. Through one calamity after another, he missed the appointment with the psychiatrist twice and was refused another appointment. We were no further ahead, and I was starting to worry. Time and again, I would painstakingly write out detailed referral letters in an attempt to seek help, and time and time again, we would face setbacks. Yet, we persevered. Was this patient derailing my attempts to help him? I did not know. But I kept going, as I did not know what else to do.

Just when it seemed as though there was nowhere else to turn, we ultimately started to clear some of the hurdles. Or so it seemed, for a while. We found an internist who addressed numerous issues and made arrangements for further testing. One step forward. But Arun's insurance company refused payment for massage and aromatherapy treatment, both of which were actually helping. One step backwards. Some people just seem to have too much bad luck. We found yet another psychiatrist. He didn't work out. Another step backwards. We found a psychologist. He seemed to be a perfect fit. The insurance company, again, didn't want to pay.

Each step of the way we were encountering not just roadblocks but also strong forces pushing us back. The frustration was building for both of us. Arun saw little progress, and I felt as though I was running out of options. I wondered if he was beginning to lose faith in me. It seemed as though each time we got a good idea or found a treatment that seemed to be providing benefit, somehow it became inaccessible. Sigh. We shared those together – sighs of despair and frustration.

Together we also shared the frustrations of minor irritants that all ultimately affected his suffering. I wondered where we would turn next, but I tried to hide my fear and concern from this man who was desperately hoping that I would be able to help alleviate some of his suffering. I was even more convinced than ever before that medical school had not prepared me for situations like this, nor had my residency. I felt my despair growing as my trusting patient became more and more desolate. Yet I persevered.

But then we turned the corner. Good psychologist – check. Good psychiatrist – check. And then there was me – the family doctor, who was witnessing this dramatic transformation and the joys that hope can bring to a life that has been filled with suffering. Other health care providers come and go, but we three formed the core team. And a team we were. There was no stepping on toes, and no squashing of egos. We were all working towards the best possible outcome for the patient, and Arun appreciated this. Through ups and downs, we examined the progress that he had made thus far. At some points it seemed as though there had been none, but that's when we would stop to evaluate. Wow! We had made tremendous progress. But it had been a long time coming.

Once a month, and occasionally more frequently, I saw Arun's name on my schedule. No longer did I sigh or react with fear or hesitation. I know that there would be visits focusing on the positive, and also visits where the negative would try to creep in. But progress was being made, and neither of us could deny that. The bulk of our energy focused on the continued enjoyment from the key components of Arun's life, all the while sorting through the best treatment options for his chronic illnesses. As we worked our way through maintaining the most important elements of this young man's life, I continued to witness the changes that occurred in Arun. Although he could not always see it, I continued to witness his tremendous change. Slowly I saw growth. Insight bloomed, and his determination increased. What an honor to share in that transformation.

This case highlights some salient features of the patient-doctor relationship. First and foremost is the temporal nature of this relationship. While thorough histories are important at the outset, the relationship develops over time, similar to any other relationship between two individuals. The roles and responsibilities of the parties involved are shaped through shared experiences. Through my interactions with Arun, I have gained an appreciation of the importance of addressing not only the disease (or diseases, as the case may be), but also of focusing on the individual's illness experience. While physical well-being may present more of a challenge, together with this patient, I have also addressed the social, emotional and spiritual aspects of his health. Working on all the aspects of his health and making small changes in each, I have gradually achieved a greater appreciation of the whole person, and in doing so, have diminished the suffering of the person as a whole.

48 The Heartsink Patient

Hugh Hindle and Judith Belle Brown

Outside the wind howled relentlessly. As I glanced out my office window, the snow pelted to the ground, heralding the entrance to the holiday season. Leona's name stood at the top of my patient list for the day. Historically, seeing her name would have prompted an inner sigh as I anticipated my encounter with this "heartsink" patient. But this was no longer the case; I now welcomed her visits on some level.

December was always a bad time of year for Leona, and she needed a little more support than usual to help her manage her "nerves." At times her agitation was apparent, as she sat with her knees shaking uncontrollably. "Can I take a few more Ativan?" she would ask. Her depression had also been worse this year, compounded by her worry and frustration about her mother, who had always been rather dependent on Leona and showed early signs of dementia. "She can't even go to the store to pick up her prescriptions. My brothers say I should do less and they will help out, but they're not living here," Leona stated resentfully. She then reminded me that she would be 61 in a week's time. This appeared to be contributing to her low mood as well.

At this visit, we didn't talk about Leona's general body pain. Neither of us quite knew what the root of her pain syndrome was, although Leona believed that her osteoporosis was at least partly to blame. She had experienced pain for so long, it didn't seem profitable to discuss it directly.

Leona had spent most of her life in our small town. She moved here as a child, and her father was very much the dominant figure from her childhood. Although he did not drink, he was given to episodes of rage and tolerated no arguments. Her mother was a passive person, who always acquiesced to the head of the family. Leona was the only girl and had four younger brothers. She was regarded as the "bad child" and suffered frequent abusive verbal tirades. When Leona was 15, she was charged after several episodes of shoplifting and petty theft. She was sent away to a juvenile institution in "the big city" and was not allowed to return home when it became apparent that she was pregnant. Instead, Leona was transferred to a home for "unwed mothers" run by a religious order until her baby was born. Her father decided "it" would be adopted, and that was the end of the matter. Leona returned home, where nobody ever discussed her pregnancy or the baby. Although her father died many years ago, Leona's resentment still simmered barely below the surface.

In her early 20s she married an abusive, alcoholic man and had to flee the marriage after a few years. Leona never became pregnant again. Although she trained as a secretary, she didn't enjoy the job and always worked as a waitress. She hasn't been able to work since her pancreatitis and is now supported by a disability pension. The resulting income was meager, so she gave up her own apartment and moved in with her widowed mother. Her youngest brother had now taken on the role of the autocratic father. At a recent family conference to discuss possible long-term care for their mother, he called Leona "stupid." Leona couldn't even get angry; she just became mute.

Leona had been as unfortunate in medicine as she had been in life. She suffered for years with depression, hypertension, chronic bone and muscle pain, and migraines. Her migraines improved when she had a hysterectomy for chronic pelvic pain 18 years ago, but her body pain didn't. A few years later I thought I had explained her abdominal pain when investigations showed a large but non-malignant gastric ulcer. Partial gastrectomy traded her abdominal pain for persistent nausea. The rest of her body still hurt.

Next she had a dreadful episode of pancreatitis and spent months in ICU. Leona survived, but she lost her spleen and all of her large bowel, leaving her with an ileostomy and a tendency towards recurrent bowel obstructions. Over time she slowly recovered and regained weight to her usual 85 pounds, only to drive into a lamppost, breaking her femur and pelvis and losing the sight in one eye. Her blind eye was sutured closed – combined with her skeletal frame, this gave her a rather startling appearance.

Two good things had happened medically for her this year. She had a cataract removed, with much anxiety, from her "good" eye; subsequently the ophthalmologist unstuck the lid of her bad eye. Both procedures went extremely well.

Despite the litany of medical tragedy, Leona only looked about 50 and walked without a limp. She managed her ileostomy totally independently and without fuss. However, she was rather stooped and very thin. Her skin was frequently scratched from dealings with her cat, and the front of her hair was often singed from cigarette burns. Leona told me it was because of the way she held her cigarettes, but I had a persistent image of her awakening to the smell of charring hair.

I have seen Leona as a patient for the last 20 years, and I probably saw her at least once a month over that time. Most of the visits were ritualistic, involving taking blood pressure and refilling prescriptions, but no real "therapy" of consequence. Leona was generally seeking permission to take even more psychotropic medication, and I have tried to put a lid on the benzodiazepine consumption. Leona never argued; that's not how you behaved around men.

Every December our visits became more intense. We share a birthday on New Year's Eve. Leona's birthday was not a happy time. Her baby was born on December 30th and removed from her on her 16th birthday. I am almost exactly a year older than her baby. She had spent several years trying to get in touch with her son, but all she knew was that he was adopted by a lawyer and his wife. The only memento she had was a photo of him at six months of age. She brought the photo in to show me at her last visit, but she wouldn't look at it. There was no hope that she would ever know her son.

Over the years, Leona and I developed a relationship that worked for us. When we started, visits were the classic "heartsink" pattern, with lots of physical symptoms, obvious psychosocial distress and no ability to develop a common plan. I dreaded her monthly appointment and would often keep her waiting while I made a phone call or had a coffee. I was stuck trying to make a diagnosis of the cause of her pains. I seemed to have the choice of either rejecting her symptoms by responding "I don't think your headaches are severe enough to warrant Demerol" or colluding with her untenable diagnosis in a conspiratorial tone: "Yes, I think it is the osteoporosis that is making your shoulder blades so sore." The key to making progress seemed to have been developing an understanding and a respect for Leona as a person.

We have slowly chipped away at the problems, and together Leona and I now generally feel comfortable without a biomedical explanation for her multiple pains. She talks less about her pain and more about her sadness and the many challenges throughout her life. We think of her life in terms of all her losses, and just "getting by" becomes an admirable goal, given the financial and social poverty of her life. Our working together relies on 20 years of mutual history held together by trust and respect.

As Leona prepares to leave the office, I look out the window again. The wind has died down, the snow has ceased and sun is slowly peaking through the clouds.

49 A Case in Complexity – Part 1

Susan Woolhouse, Tanya Thornton and Judith Belle Brown

Bob sauntered into the exam room, eased his lean, unkempt frame into the chair and announced, "Doc, you don't look a day out of high school! I'm really complicated. I'm probably too complicated for you."

As I had only been in practice one week, it merely took a split second for me to agree, "You're probably right. You may indeed be complicated and I may look young, but I think I can still help you if you are willing to let me try."

"Well, we'll just have to wait and see," he grumbled. "Just sort me out, and renew my diabetic meds and I'll be out of your hair."

"Okay, what needs to be sorted out?"

"Well, I can't afford to live in the apartment any longer since Gerry moved out. I can barely pay for my meds, now that I have to pay the rent on my own. Besides, I don't even know if I want to live there anymore – it's not the safest place in town you know."

I wasn't trained in medical school to find people housing. The meds – *that* I can do. I flipped through his scant chart: 53 years old, type 2 diabetes for 10 years, poorly controlled due to social circumstances. I learned that Bob had spent 20 years living in prison and, upon release, was living in a run-down rooming house and not taking any insulin. This precipitated a myocardial infarction and a lengthy hospitalization whereby, upon discharge, he started to receive more regular care at our inner-city medical clinic. Since then, his HgA1c had improved remarkably and his renal status and lipid profile had normalized.

"Hey doc, you there? I'm still sitting here waiting for my meds."

"Oh sorry, I was just familiarizing myself with your past medical history."

"Well, if you had just asked me, I could have told you and saved us both the time. I have no money, other than what little disability provides, I have no friends, I haven't been out long enough for any 'socialization,' my family left me when I was put in the can. And, as I said, my place ain't exactly the Ritz. I have a couple of deadbolts on the door, but that wouldn't stop them if they wanted to get in."

Bob lived in constant fear with a nonexistent support system. It was that first day with Bob that I realized how modifying my expectations and hoping for small victories were the key to maintaining my sanity and ultimately providing good patient care, regardless if I knew nothing about how to find a person adequate housing.

"How much insulin are you on?"

"Thirty-five units in the morning and 20 units at night."

"That's a lot of insulin. Do you –"

"Listen, that's what the specialist in hospital put me on, that's what I take, that's what I need renewed. That's all. You able to do that?" Bob challenged.

"Sure, I just wanted to make sure that you aren't getting any low numbers; any blood sugars less than four?"

"Not many, but a few."

"Do you have your glucometer book?"

"Of course I do." Bob retorted. He pulled out his log book from the worn pack he carried slung across his torso.

As I scanned through his log, I realized that Bob was not as he appeared. Although unshaven and in stained clothing, he maintained a meticulous record of his blood sugars, usually checking them four times a day. Unfortunately, more than a quarter of his readings were in the hypoglycemic range. "I'm worried about all these numbers less than four. How do you feel when they are that low?"

"A bit shaky I guess. But I don't want another heart attack!"

"Agreed. I don't want that for you either, but these lows are too risky for you. How about food – do you have enough money to eat appropriately?"

"What the hell is 'eating appropriately'? Listen, as I told you, I barely got enough money for meds and rent, let alone 'appropriate food,'" he scoffed, almost spitting out the words. "I count the carbohydrates as they said I should in hospital, I record it all." With that, he started rooting through his sack again and produced another record of precise calorie and carbohydrate counts.

"Wow, this is impressive." I congratulated, trying to regain the ground I was rapidly losing in relationship building. "I wonder if the dietician and social worker at our clinic would be able to put you in touch with some community resources that would help you better access the food you need to prevent you from getting so many lows." As I thought aloud, his demeanor that challenged everything I suggested softened.

"You think you can get me some food? Good healthy stuff?"

"Yeah, maybe."

"Okay. What about my place?"

"Well, to be honest Bob, I don't know much about finding housing." I paused, then added, "But I can ask around."

"Well that's all I ask – that you be upfront with me. I told you I was complicated."

"Yes you did," I conceded.

Bob took the scripts. Although he refused to lower the dosages of his insulin, he made appointments to see both the dietician and social worker the following week. As Bob had not been receiving medical care until recently, simply attending regular appointments with the team, with whom he felt safe, was an unspoken priority for me.

He returned for follow-up diabetic care, and the more opinions I gave about management, the more he challenged my credentials. I would say one thing and he would do the opposite.

Then one day, amid quibbles over smoking, he began to share – not his opinions, but his story. I sat speechless, listening attentively. Our eyes locked. His voice softened and he talked and talked and talked. Where had this come from? Was this the same argumentative soul who gave me heart-sink at our monthly visits? The more I heard Bob's story, the more I understood the context of his illness. I became cognizant of his need for control. I learned that he had suffered a life plagued by severe mental health challenges, including chronic symptoms of anxiety, poor sleep, social phobia and flashbacks. He dealt with his trauma-induced anxiety by dissociating himself. At times when he was being physically and sexually assaulted as a child, he simply "froze" and "disconnected." He had spent his life being told what to do – often in ways that were brutal and violent. Bob felt disdain for anyone in a position of power. This included health care providers – and me. I suddenly grasped why he questioned my knowledge and decisions. I needed to back off and stop taking his vitriol personally.

As I pondered these things, his voice interrupted my thoughts. "Hey doc, you still there?" He was waving his hand in front of my face.

"Yes, Bob. I – I, I didn't realize any of this."

"Well of course you didn't, you never asked."

"That's true." We sat silent for a moment. Something had changed between us. He had exposed his ghosts – to me. In that moment, I realized that he trusted me. "Bob, have you shared this with anyone else?"

"No, I've been in the can – remember. And besides, who wants to hear my sob story?"

"I think I know of someone who not only would like to hear it, but could help you." I paused to gauge his reaction. "Would you meet with the psychiatrist at the center? If you don't feel comfortable with him, you can always leave or not return for follow-up, but I think you might be surprised by his willing ear."

"Okay. Only if you think it might help. But if I don't like him, I'm outta there."

"It's a deal."

Bob was finally diagnosed with complex post-traumatic stress disorder. Through our interactions, I learned about countertransference firsthand and how to check these feelings at the door. I began to realize how significant our relationship was to Bob. He had finally found a place that was safe and predictable. Furthermore, his visits served as a useful outlet to vent his frustrations and feelings. A small victory!

Bob expected me to listen to his ideas about management and, above all, be open and honest with him when I didn't know the answers. Just as Bob felt overwhelmed with his situation, it was easy for me, his inexperienced provider, to often feel engulfed and inadequate. I came to learn how to recognize these reactions within myself and how to use them to be forthright with Bob – because ultimately, that's all he hoped for.

50 A Case in Complexity – Part 2

Susan Woolhouse, Tanya Thornton and Judith Belle Brown

"Doc, I just wanted to show you that I was right and you were wrong," Bob said, smiling. He had just handed me a pamphlet about diabetes that "contradicted" my advice from a previous visit.

I read the information and smiled. "Bob, sometimes we'll have to agree to disagree. But in the end, you're the boss, okay?"

Bob just continued to smile. This was a new development – my concessions and his smiles. We were breaking new ground in the relationship. We were learning together: how to form new ways of finding common ground. It wasn't always easy. One of the barriers to finding common ground was my reaction to having my "authority" questioned. This was especially difficult when I had little experience to rely upon and thus felt my confidence wane.

As time passed and our relationship evolved, Bob and I formed a deeper understanding of our unique roles. Mine was to secure a safe, consistent place, his was to show up and share. When caring for marginalized populations, forming a trusting relationship is paramount. While the foundation of the relationship was being formed, the focus was on providing a context of trust, so that Bob would return for follow-up care. One of the factors that facilitated this trust was the creation of a safe space. I learned to be attentive at all times, actively present. I zoned-out less and listened more. By simply being present, I hoped to send Bob a message that I cared for him and would not abandon him. This tenuous time in our relationship was the "testing period." His cantankerous control, which permeated the visits, at times was a façade and at times the outward manifestation of his complex soul. Yes, he was complex. He was right about that.

With the development of trust and a stronger patient-physician relationship, I began to feel less overwhelmed, and my confidence increased. As a result, I was better able to attend to Bob's needs, which in turn further strengthened our relationship and fostered our finding of common ground.

Finding common ground is as unique as each illness experience. It seemed more challenging when it came to Bob's diabetes. He had very peculiar notions about his diet and insulin. I questioned many of these, particularly since one of my concerns was his low weight and his low-calorie diet, which led to frequent episodes of hypoglycemia.

While Bob had allowed the clinic social worker to hook him up with the local food bank, I continued to be concerned about the quality of his diet.

"Are you able to get the necessary food you need at the food bank?" I inquired of Bob.

"There you go again, doc, 'necessary food,' 'appropriate food'! What I get is what I can cook on the hotplate at the rooming house," retorted Bob.

"Right, right," I responded sheepishly. Bob's housing dilemma remained unsolved and continued to be a major aggravation for him.

I had previously tried to connect Bob with the dietician and the social worker at the clinic. But he had been very reluctant to accept their assistance on an ongoing basis. However, I decided to once again introduce the possibility of their involvement.

"What about meeting with the social worker to talk about the option of subsidized housing?" I asked tentatively.

"Those government-run places?" Bob replied incredulously. "No way I'm going to live in one of those with all their rules and regulations! I just got my freedom back after 20 years in the joint and no one is telling me what to do now!"

Once again, I hit a roadblock with Bob. I had to admit to myself that perhaps it was my own doing – I failed to be sensitive to his complex past.

"Okay, I think I understand now where you are coming from Bob. How about I sit down with the social worker and we brainstorm other options before I see you next week?"

"Now you're talkin' doc!" Bob said heartily, giving me a slap on my back as he stood to leave.

Finding common ground with respect to Bob's mental health was less of a struggle. To his surprise, he connected with the psychiatrist. After starting on an antidepressant, his symptoms of anxiety and social phobia decreased. This in turn enabled him to access more supports for his mental health. The social worker referred Bob to a mental health outreach organization, which did home visits and arranged social activities in the community. Bob's vigilance about his diabetes self-management continued – that was part of who he was – but it caused less anxiety for him and for me. Part of this was facilitated by Bob's attendance at group sessions conducted by the diabetes educator.

"Those group meetings are real fine, doc," Bob said, smirking sarcastically.

He had been, as I anticipated, reticent to attend. Nevertheless, the experience had been not only educational, but also served as another social outlet for this isolated man.

Malnutrition, inadequate housing, and social isolation had initially contributed to a general failure to thrive and extreme loneliness. The team's approach to improve his whole health, including his context, became empowering for him and enhanced his overall well-being. Bob's life had changed, albeit slowly. Patience, trust and respect fostered our relationship. I began to learn who Bob really was and at how I could help him beyond glycemic control. Although I never did learn how to find affordable housing for him, he accepted this as part of my limitations, and somehow it fostered our bond.

Continuing to be present, to listen and to advocate for Bob were core tenets of his care. We did not always see eye to eye with regards to his diabetes management, but I continue to assure him I would remain steadfast. He made tremendous gains – as did I. He had tested me, and I had passed. It was my responsibility to maintain the grade.

References

Balint M. *The Doctor, His Patient, and the Illness*. New York, NY: International Universities Press; 1957.

Belenky MF, Clinchy BM, Goldberger NR, *et al. Women's Ways of Knowing: the development of self, voice, and mind*. New York, NY: Basic Books; 1986.

Borkan JM. Examining American family medicine in the new world order: a study of five practices. *J Fam Pract*. 1999; **48**(8): 6207.

Bowen M. Theory in the practice of psychotherapy. In: Guerin PJ, editor. *Family Therapy: theory and practice*. New York, NY: Gardner Press; 1976.

Bowen M. Toward the differentiation of self in one's family of origin. In: Bowen M, editor. *Family Therapy in Clinical Practice*. New York, NY: Jason Aronson; 1978.

Bowlby J. *Attachment and Loss: vol. 2, Separation: anxiety and anger*. New York, NY: Basic Books; 1973.

Bowlby J. *Attachment and Loss: vol. 1, Attachment*. New York, NY: Basic Books; 1982.

Broderick P, Blewitt P. *The Life Span: human development for helping professionals*. 3rd edition. New Jersey: Merrill-Prentice Hall; 2010.

Brown JB, Stewart M, Weston WW. *Challenges and Solutions in Patient-Centered Care: a case book*. Oxford: Radcliffe Medical Press; 2002.

Cameron IA. The importance of stories. *Can Fam Physician*. 2011; **57**(1): 66–7.

Candib LM. Ways of knowing in family medicine: contributions from a feminist perspective. *Fam Med*. 1988; **20**(2): 133–6.

Cassell EJ. *The Nature of Suffering and the Goals of Medicine*. New York, NY: Oxford University Press; 1991.

Charon R. Narrative and Medicine. *NEJM*. 2004; **350**(9): 862–4.

Charon R. *Narrative Medicine: honoring the stories of illness*. Oxford: Oxford University Press; 2006.

Charon R. What to do with stories: the sciences of narrative medicine. *Can Fam Physician*. 2007; **53**(8): 1265–7.

Cooper AF. Whose illness is it anyway? Why patient perceptions matter. *Int J Clin Pract*. 1998; **52**(8): 551–6.

de Leeuw E. Concepts in health promotion: the notion of relativism. *Soc Sci Med*. 1989; **29**(11): 1281–8.

Dubovsky SL. *Psychotherapeutics in Primary Care*. New York, NY: Grune and Stratton; 1981.

Edwards A, Elwyn G, editors. *Shared Decision-Making in Health Care – Achieving Evidence-Based Patient Choice*. 2nd edition. Oxford: Oxford University Press; 2009.

Epstein RM. Mindful practice. *JAMA*. 1999; **282**(9): 833–9.

Epstein RM, Franks P, Shields CG, *et al*. Patient-centered communication and diagnostic testing. *Ann Fam Med*. 2005; **3**(5): 415–21.

Epstein RM, Campbell TL, Cohen-Cole SA, *et al*. Perspectives on patient-doctor communication. *J Fam Pract*. 1993; **37**(4): 377–88.

Erikson EH. *Childhood and Society*. New York, NY: WW Norton & Company; 1950.

Erikson EH. *The Life Cycle Completed: a review*. New York, NY: WW Norton & Company; 1982.

Fossum B, Arborelius E. Patient-centered communication: videotaped consultations. *Patient Educ Couns*. 2004; **54**(2): 163–9.

Frank AW. *The Wounded Storyteller: body, illness and ethics*. Chicago, IL: University of Chicago Press; 1995.

Frank AW. *The Renewal of Generosity: illness, medicine and how to live*. Chicago, IL: University of Chicago Press; 2004.

Goldberg PE. The physician-patient relationship: three psychodynamic concepts that can be applied to primary care. *Arch Fam Med*. 2000; **9**(10): 116–48.

Golin CE, DiMatteo MR, Gelberg L. The role of patient participation in the doctor visit. Implications for adherence to diabetes care. *Diabetes Care*. 1996; **19**(10): 1153–64.

Gorman E. Chronic degenerative conditions, disability and loss. In: Harris DL, editor. *Counting Our Losses: reflecting on change, loss and transition in everyday life*. New York, NY: Routledge; 2011.

Greenfield S, Kaplan SH, Ware JE Jr, *et al*. Patients' participation in medical care: effects on blood sugar control and quality of life in diabetes. *J Gen Intern Med*. 1988; **3**(5): 448–57.

Greenhalgh T, Hurwitz B. *Narrative Based Medicine: dialogue and discourse in clinical practice*. London: BMJ Books; 1998.

Griffin SJ, Kinmonth AL, Veltman MW, *et al*. Effect on health-related outcomes of interventions to alter the interaction between patients and practitioners: a systematic review of trials. *Ann Fam Med*. 2004; **2**(6): 595–608.

Groopman J. *How Doctors Think*. Boston, MA: Houghton Mifflin Company; 2008.

Guest A. *Taking Sides: clashing views in lifespan development*. Dubuque, IA: McGraw-Hill; 2007.

Harris DL. *Counting Our Losses: reflecting on change, loss and transition in everyday life*. New York, NY: Routledge; 2011.

Harris DL. Infertility and reproductive loss. In: Harris, 2011, op. cit.

Haug M, Lavin B. *Consumerism in Medicine: challenging physician authority*. Beverly Hills, CA: Sage; 1983.

Helman CG. *Culture, Health and Illness*. 4th edition. London: Arnold; 2007.

Hurowitz JC. Toward a social policy for health. *NEJM*. 1993; **329**(2): 130–3.

Jordan JV, Kaplan AG, Miller JB, *et al*. *Women's Growth in Connection: writings from the Stone Center*. New York, NY: The Guilford Press; 1991.

Juckett G. Cross-cultural medicine. *Am Fam Physician*. 2005; **72**(11): 2267–74.

Kaplan SH, Greenfields S, Ware JE Jr. Assessing the effects of physician-patient interactions on the outcomes of chronic disease. *Med Care.* 1989; **27**(3 Suppl.): S110–27.

Kleinman AL, Eisenberg L, Good B. Culture, illness, and care: clinical lessons from anthropologic and cross-cultural research. *Ann Int Med.* 1978; **88**(2): 251–8.

Kon AA. The shared decision-making continuum. *JAMA.* 2010; **304**(8): 903–4.

Krupat E, Rosenkranz SL, Yeager CM, *et al.* The practice orientations of physicians and patients: the effect of doctors-patient congruence on satisfaction. *Patient Educ Couns.* 2000; **39**(1): 49–59.

Lang F, Floyd MR, Beine KL. Clues to patients' explanations and concerns about their illnesses. *Arch Fam Med.* 2000; **9**(3): 222–7.

Lantos J, Matlock AM, Wendler D. Clinician integrity and limits to patient autonomy. *JAMA.* 2011; **305**(5): 495–9.

Loxtercamp D. Being there: on the place of the family physician. *J Am Board Fam Pract.* 1991; **4**(5): 354–60.

Loxtercamp D. A vow of connectedness: views from the road to Beaver's farm. *Fam Med.* 2001; **33**(4): 244–7.

Malterud K. Key questions – a strategy for modifying clinical communication. Transforming tacit skills into a clinical method. *Scand J Prim Health Care.* 1994; **12**(2): 121–7.

Mayeroff M. *On Caring.* New York, NY: Harper & Row; 1972.

McDaniel S, Campbell TL, Seaburn DB. *Family-Oriented Primary Care: a manual for medical providers.* New York, NY: Springer-Verlag; 1990.

McWilliam CL, Stewart M, Brown JB, *et al.* Creating empowering meaning: an interactive process of promoting health with chronically ill older persons. *Health Promotion International.* 1997; **14**(1): 27–41.

Mishler EG. *Discourse of Medicine: dialectics of medical interviews.* Norwood, NJ: Ablex; 1984.

Montgomery CL. *Healing Through Communication: the practice of caring.* Newbury Park, CA: Sage; 1993.

Novack DH, Suchman AL, Clark W, *et al.* Calibrating the physician. Personal awareness and effective patient care. *JAMA.* 1997; **278**(6): 502–9.

Nulan S. *The Soul of Medicine.* New York, NY: Kaplan Publishing; 2010.

Ofri D. *Incidental Findings: lesson from my patients in the art of medicine.* Boston, MA: Beacon Press; 2005.

Quill TE, Brody H. Physician recommendations and patient autonomy: finding a balance between physician power and patient choice. *Ann Int Med.* 1996; **125**(9): 763–9.

Pories S, Jain S, Harper G. *The Soul of a Doctor.* Chapel Hill, NC: Algonquin Books of Chapel Hill; 2006.

Pottie K, Brown JB, Dunn S. The resettlement of Central American men in Canada: from emotional distress to successful integration. *Refuge.* 2005; **22**(2): 101–11.

Pullen D, Lonie C, Cam D, *et al.* Medical care of doctors. *Med J Aust.* 1995; **162**(9): 481–4.

Ransom D. The family in family medicine: reflections on the first 25 years. *Family Systems Med.* 1993; **11**(1): 25–9.

Rao JK, Anderson LA, Inui TS, *et al.* Communication interventions make a difference in conversations between physicians and patients: a systematic review of the evidence. *Med Care.* 2007; **45**(4): 340–9.

Redelmeier DA, Molin JP, Tibshirani RJ. A randomized trial of compassionate care for the homeless in an emergency department. *Lancet.* 1995; **345**(8958): 1131–4.

Rogers C. Significant learning. In: Rogers C, editor. *On Becoming a Person.* Boston, MA: Houghton Mifflin; 1961.

Rolland J. Chronic illness and the family life cycle. In: Carter B, McGoldrick M, editors. *The Changing Family Life Cycle: a framework for family therapy.* Boston, MA: Allyn and Bacon; 1989.

Rosenberg E, Xenocostas S, Dao M, *et al.* GPs' strategies in intercultural clinical encounters. *Fam Pract.* 2007; **24**(2): 145–51.

Roter D, Hall J. *Improving Psychosocial Problem Address in Primary Care: is it possible and what difference does it make?* Toronto: The International Consensus Conference on Doctor-Patient Communication; 1992.

Santrock J. *A Topical Approach to Life-Span Development.* New York, NY: McGraw-Hill; 2007.

Sawicki W. We are not like other people: identity loss and reconstruction following migration. In: Harris, 2011, op. cit.

Scarf M. *Intimate Worlds: life inside the family.* New York, NY: Random House; 1995.

Schriver J. *Human Behavior and the Social Environment.* 4th edition. New York, NY: Pearson; 2004.

Searight HR, Gafford J. Cultural diversity at the end of life: issues and guidelines for family physicians. *Am Fam Physician.* 2005; **71**(3): 515–22.

Stachtchenko S, Jenicek M. Conceptual differences between prevention and health promotion: research implications for community health programs. *Can J Public Health.* 1990; **81**(8): 53–9.

Stein HF. What is therapeutic in clinical relationships? *Fam Med.* 1985; **17**(5): 188–94.

Stewart M, Roter D. *Communicating with Medical Patients.* Newbury Park, CA: Sage; 1989.

Stewart M, Brown JB, Boon H, *et al.* Evidence on patient-doctor communication. *Cancer Prev Control.* 1999; **3**(1): 25–30.

Stewart M, Brown JB, Weston WW, *et al. Patient-Centered Medicine: transforming the clinical method.* 2nd edition. Oxford: Radcliffe Medical Press; 2003.

Stewart M, Brown JB, Hammerton J, *et al.* Improving communication between doctors and breast cancer patients. *Ann Fam Med.* 2007; **5**(5): 387–94.

Stewart M, Ryan BL, Bodea C. Is patient-centred care associated with lower diagnostic costs? *Healthcare Policy.* 2011; **6**(4): 27–31.

Suchman AL, Matthews DA. What makes the patient-doctor relationship therapeutic? Exploring the connexional dimension of medical care. *Ann Intern Med.* 1988; **108**(1): 125–30.

Szasz TS, Hollender MH. The basic model of the doctor-patient relationship. *AMA Arch Intern Med.* 1956; **97**(5): 585–92.

Thorsen H, Witt K, Hollnagel H, *et al.* The purpose of the general practice consultation from the patient's perspective – theoretical aspects. *Fam Pract.* 2001; **18**(6): 638–43.

Trevalon M, Murray-Garcia J. Cultural humility versus cultural competence: a critical distinction in defining physician training outcomes in multicultural education. *J Health Care Poor Underserved.* 1998; **9**(2): 117–25.

Tuckett D, Boulton M, Olson C, *et al. Meetings Between Experts: an approach to sharing ideas in medical consultations.* New York, NY: Tavistock; 1985.

Vaillant GE. Positive emotions, spirituality and the practice of psychiatry. *Mental Health, Spirituality, Mind.* 2008; **6**(1): 48–62.

Veatch R. Models for ethical medicine in a revolutionary age. *Hastings Cent Rep.* 1972; **2**(3): 5–7.

Watson J. *Nursing: human science and human care.* New York, NY: Appleton-Century-Crofts; 1985.

Wood ML. Naming the illness: the power of words. *Fam Med.* 1991; **23**(7): 534–8.

Woods ME, Hollis F. *Casework: a psychosocial therapy.* New York, NY: McGraw-Hill; 1990.

Woolhouse S, Brown JB, Thind A. 'Meeting people where they're at': experiences of family physicians engaging women who use illicit drugs. *Ann Fam Med.* 2011; **9**(3): 244–9.

World Health Organization. Health promotion: a discussion document on the concept and principles. *Health Promot Int.* 1986; **1**(1): 73–6.

Index